The Jossey-Bass/AHA Press Series translates the latest ideas on health care management into practical and actionable terms. Together, Jossey-Bass and the American Hospital Association offer these essential resources for the health care leaders of today and tomorrow.

The CEO's Guide to Health Care Information Systems

Second Edition

JOSEPH M. DeLUCA
REBECCA ENMARK

JOSSEY-BASS
A Wiley Company
San Francisco

Health Forum, Inc.
An American Hospital Association Company
CHICAGO press

Library of Congress Cataloging-in-Publication Data
DeLuca, Joseph M., 1956–
  The CEO's guide to health care information systems / Joseph M. DeLuca, Rebecca Enmark. — 2nd ed.
    p. cm. — (The Jossey-Bass/AHA Press series)
  Includes index.
  ISBN 0-7879-5277-X (pb.:alk. paper)
    1. Health services administration—Data processing. 2. Information storage and retrieval systems—Medical care. I. Cagan, Rebecca Enmark. II. Title. III. Series.

RA971.6D45 2001
362.1'0285—dc21   2001025893

SECOND EDITION
PB Printing   10 9 8 7 6 5 4 3 2

CONTENTS

List of Figures, Tables, and Exhibits   vii

About the Authors   ix

Preface   xi

Acknowledgments   xv

1. **Health Care Information Technology**   1

2. **Information Systems Features and Functions**   27

3. **The Integrated Delivery System**   59

4. **The Systems Life Cycle**   83

5. **Managing Health Care Information Technology**   111

    Appendix: Technology Concepts   135

    Glossary   143

    Index   157

LIST OF FIGURES, TABLES, AND EXHIBITS

FIGURES

Figure 2.1	Internet-Intranet-Extranet Systems Architecture	31
Figure 2.2	Return-on-Investment Expectations	53
Figure 2.3	Benefit Mapping	57
Figure 3.1	Affiliation IDS Model	67
Figure 3.2	Regional Delivery IDS Model	69
Figure 3.3	Affiliation with Central Services IDS Model	70
Figure 3.4	Corporate Ownership IDS Model	71
Figure 4.1	Business to Technology Alignment Methodology	85
Figure 4.2	Value-Based Systems and Processes	92

TABLES

Table 1.1	Health Care Application Systems	10
Table 1.2	Health Care Foundation and Advanced Technologies	12
Table 1.3	Comparison of Information Technology Market Providers	19
Table 2.1	Patient Administration and Management Systems	33
Table 2.2	General Financial Management Systems	34
Table 2.3	Physician Practice Management Systems	35
Table 2.4	Home Health Systems	36

Table 2.5	Financial Decision Support Systems	39
Table 2.6	Clinical Decision Support Systems	40
Table 2.7	General Clinical, Ancillary, and Specialty Site Systems	42
Table 2.8	Medical Management Systems	43
Table 2.9	Electronic Medical Records	44
Table 2.10	Managed Care Systems	46
Table 2.11	Enterprise Systems	48
Table 2.12	Consumer Health Systems	50
Table 2.13	Advanced Technologies	51
Table 2.14	Patient Scheduling Data Exchanges	54
Table 2.15	Investment Benefits	56
Table 3.1	Five Integration Areas	63
Table 3.2	Key IDS Applications and Focus	64
Table 3.3	IDS Model Summary	74
Table 4.1	Life Cycle Considerations	90
Table 4.2	Sample Contract Issues Document	107
Table 5.1	The Role of the Chief Information Officer	113
Table 5.2	Situational Governance	121

EXHIBITS

Exhibit 3.1	Components of Integration	61
Exhibit 4.1	IT Planning Process Milestones	95
Exhibit 4.2	Choosing a Data Collection Tool	99
Exhibit 4.3	Typical Contents of a Vendor System Proposal	101
Exhibit 4.4	Phases of Information Technology Contracting	103
Exhibit 4.5	Components of a System Implementation Plan	109
Exhibit 5.1	Small Delivery Systems	123
Exhibit 5.2	Sample Central Service Organization Structure and Responsibilities	124

ABOUT THE AUTHORS

Joseph M. DeLuca, chief executive officer of Information Technology Optimizers (a business unit of Health Care Investment Visions LLC), is a health care information technology futurist, bringing innovative wisdom and practical experience to both the health care and information technology market segments. DeLuca works closely with health care providers, payers, and public policy and research organizations, as well as with health care IT entrepreneurs, developers, suppliers, and financiers. His unique perspective and knowledge have evolved over two decades of providing successful advisory services for his clients.

A fellow in the American College of Healthcare Executives (FACHE), DeLuca earned his master of arts degree in health services administration at the University of Wisconsin at Madison and his bachelor of arts degree in biology, magna cum laude, at Lawrence University in Appleton, Wisconsin. He is a frequent speaker at regional and national conferences and is widely published on health care and information technology topics.

Rebecca Enmark, research director of Health Care Investment Visions LLC, studies health care market, technology, and company behaviors. Over the course of her career, she has worked closely with health care provider and technology organizations to focus IT planning, use, and development in support of short- and long-term business and market requirements. Enmark holds a master's degree in library and information studies and a bachelor of arts in English literature, both from the University of California at Berkeley. She has published widely on information technology topics in industry journals and monographs.

PREFACE

The application of information technology (IT) in our daily life is already providing immense gains in personal knowledge, economic productivity, and human creativity. Future advances in IT will accelerate the value of human-computer interaction far beyond what we can imagine today, at a pace and intensity that will continue to challenge our cultural, geopolitical, social, and legal systems. Indeed, the differences that exist between the human dimension and the computer are narrowing rapidly. Advances in voice- and thought-based computer command systems, neural-network computers, robotics, genomic-based information systems, nano-information technologies, and molecular computing are closing the gap between humans and machines.

Our health care system is not, and indeed should not be, excluded from these vigorous trends. Nationally, our heath care financing and delivery system is in a state of flux—some would say chaos. Local markets remain—and rightly so, in the eyes of many—the nexus of control over health care supply, demand, delivery, financing, and pricing. Recent technology advances in electronic commerce and e-health have created expectations of capability and instant participation by citizen, consumer, patient, and care provider constituencies in the health care process. These expectations will only expand over time.

Information system capabilities within our payer and provider systems remain a conundrum to many people. The world outside of health care embraces new information technology applications openly, adopting a value-oriented and progressive investment philosophy. Yet most of the health care world views information technology as—at best—a necessary cost, focused on doing what has always been done in a more efficient manner. Breakthrough information technologies and their associated value are too often shunned based on a philosophy of risk aversion rather than embraced for the tremendous advances they may represent.

A progressive and hopeful minority within the health care system, however, is pursuing a realistic, practical, and measured strategic vision of information technology. Willing to accept controlled risk, embracing the fundamental changes in human existence being driven by information technologies, and demanding plausible value propositions, these health care organizations and their leaders are moving forward in bold ways. Over time, the demonstrated capabilities and success stories of these pathfinders will open the broad potential of information technology to our entire health care system.

It is within this context of progressive yet practical strategic visioning for information technology that this book is written. Our objectives are specific:

- To provide senior management with a nontechnical introduction to the major components, functions, capabilities, and life cycle stages of health care information systems

- To inform readers about current and future trends in information technology that affect the health care information system industry and structure

- To present a model for information technology visioning, planning, selection, development, implementation, and value attainment

- To introduce the information technology supplier market and associated trends

- To discuss the role and function of information technology leadership, management, organization, and issues affecting this function

The overall goal of this book is to help executives and senior management build and maintain a solid competency in information technology in their health care organizations. Based on individual and collective knowledge, this competency should support current and emerging business and medical service requirements, allow for a continuous planning and adaptation process, and be responsive to information technology advances within the health care industry as well society in general. You will enjoy the journey.

July 2001   Joseph M. DeLuca
                                                                     Alameda, California

ACKNOWLEDGMENTS

This book owes much to the wisdom of other people:

- To Owen Doyle (1942–1992), collaborator on the first (1991) version of this work, who paved the way for much of the structure and thinking that remains today. He is still missed.

- To our corporate staff, including Jane Healy, for providing expert assistance and steady guidance in many areas.

- To our clients, with special gratitude to Craig Lanway at Hill Physicians Medical Group, for allowing us to share with you many of the learning experiences that we've shared with them.

Finally, as always, we owe a large debt of gratitude to the management and staff at Health Forum (formerly American Hospital Publishing) for their endless good humor, unflappable support, and expert guidance. Richard Hill, editorial director of AHA Press, remains a driving force behind our ability to actually deliver a workable manuscript. Thank you for everything.

CHAPTER 1

Health Care Information Technology

The health care information technology boom of the 1990s will continue—and diversify—in the twenty-first century. Over the past decade, hospitals, academic medical centers, integrated delivery systems, medical groups, managed care organizations, and health plans have spent record amounts of capital and operating funds developing foundation systems and core information technology capabilities. Today, health care information technology is acknowledged as a necessary critical success factor for every provider and payer organization. To achieve marketplace success, it is now essential that management possess a core competency in the planning, design, implementation, and use of health care information technology.

Organizations that have developed this competency are poised on the brink of an incredible opportunity. With strong technology management skills, operational redesign capabilities, and functional core information systems, IT-enabled organizations can begin to create IT-driven care delivery systems capable of breakthrough gains in quality, efficacy, population management, and cost effectiveness. Consumers, employers, and payers, as they become more technology and data savvy, will expect and demand these gains.

MYTHS AND REALITIES

Competency development is a continual process, based on organizational learning models. There are a number of commonly held information technology–related myths from which all health care organizations, regardless of competency level, can continually learn.

Myth: The Internet will change everything.

Reality: It already has.

The Internet has made a profound and irreversible change in our society and in the world of health care information technology. Information can now reach any individual who is Internet-enabled, through phone lines, cable television, local area networks, or high-speed wireless technology. Certainly, the technology of the Internet will continue to evolve, making the hardware and software in use today obsolete. However, the tremendous reach, range, and maneuverability of information fundamental in the design of the Internet will continue to expand.

More significantly, the expectations created by the Internet—health information anytime, anywhere; personal participation in the care access and management process; inexpensive access to data and communications; on-line electronic commerce—will persist into future generations of technologically sophisticated citizens, enrollees, patients, care providers, and employees. Embrace these concepts openly, and use them to attain medical service and business advantage.

Myth: We cannot change physician behavior toward information technology.

Reality: You can, but it is a long-term process.

The practice of medicine remains an individual craft, passed down through a hybrid scientific-Socratic teaching process. For sustainable change to occur, and for information technology to be part of the personal practice habit of each physician, medical school education and residencies must thoroughly incorporate clinical information tools into the craft of medicine. Medical textbooks and stethoscopes will no longer suffice; a personal digital medical assistant will be essential too.

However, today physicians of all ages and practice specialties will readily adopt technologies that offer them clear and understandable value. To be sure, physicians have made great strides in recent years in accepting the importance of information technology and incorporating useful technologies into their caregiving practices. For example, access to on-line electronic and CD-ROM medical research tools is very widely accepted, encouraged, and even demanded by today's medical caregivers because it *directly assists their efforts to treat patients.*

Show a physician an information technology that will reduce practice costs, increase profitability, improve the quality of care, increase patient satisfaction, or let them go home earlier, and they will enthusiastically use the technology. Demonstrate a definitive two-year return on investment or subsidize the investment for them, and they will become committed users. To accomplish this, it remains, in the short term, the responsibility of a vested "interested" sponsor—the delivery system, hospital, payer, independent practice association (IPA), commercial venture—to assume a leadership role in IT-related physician education, planning, funding, deployment, and use efforts.

Myth: Information technology planning is a waste of time.

Reality: In rapidly evolving markets and delivery structures, information technology plans are more important than ever.

The health care delivery and financing system is, in general, under a significant amount of near-term duress. This will continue as the twin pressures of increased system demand (by aging baby boomers and their offspring) and stagnant payment rates intensify.

Complementing this perspective, the tremendous range of information technology options available today, along with the rapid pace of change, offers both risks and opportunities for provider organizations. It is possible to reach new heights of care quality, productivity, and effectiveness through the support of information technology. At the same time, there are numerous IT-related temptations to lure an organization off track without the road map provided by clearly defined goals and objectives.

Only by consistently anchoring to a vision for information technology—one that supports business and medical service goals—can there be reasonable certainty that IT dollars are well spent and effective. Chapter Four discusses long-range planning in terms of planning time frames, techniques, and themes for infrastructure, core systems, clinical and population decision support systems, and strategic capabilities.

Myth: Detailed benefits analyses are prohibitively expensive.

Reality: Meaningful return-on-investment analysis is not just possible but both essential and cost effective.

Maximizing the near- and long-term return from an IT investment is a critical success requirement. Today, it is possible to accomplish relatively simple "best practice" comparisons, benchmarking studies, or detailed engineering-based ROI analyses (as the case may be) for any potential IT investment.

Unless a technology is so leading-edge that no one has yet implemented it successfully, someone knows what it can and cannot do. At a minimum, executives should seek out that information and examine the best practices of people already using the technology and then adapt or benchmark those practices to fit their own organization. In that way, health care organizations can build on the successes and learning lessons of others.

Organizations with clear, accurate information about internal time-based activity levels, volumes, and costs can conduct more detailed benefits analyses through either logic-based feasibility analyses or formal management engineering studies.

Whatever approach taken, establishing and quantifying the value that a technology investment provides should drive the prioritization and appropriate usage of limited funds.

Myth: Information technology = data systems.

Reality: Information technology encompasses a broad set of systems, applications, physical equipment, and capabilities.

Traditionally, management has defined or viewed IT in terms of existing data systems (finance, accounting, billing, laboratory, and so on). Today, information technology encompasses a wide range and variety of capabilities, including

- Traditional data systems
- Voice and telephone systems
- Private networks—local, wide, and metropolitan area networking technologies
- Public networks—Internet, broadband cellular
- Medical devices
- Integration technologies—interface engines, databases and repositories
- Assimilating technologies—interactive voice response, computer telephony integration, Internet-enabled patient and provider communication applications

Crucial to the successful use of these various information technologies is the need to incorporate them harmoniously into the planning and budgeting cycle.

> **Myth:** All of our technologies must be seamless to form an integrated delivery system.
>
> **Reality:** There are many models of integration.

Integrated delivery systems (IDSs) across the country are experimenting with and adopting various levels of service and technology integration. Some organizations are striving for uniform systems; others seek a consistent user view (drawing data from a centralized repository); still others focus on "circles of technology influence" within their networks or on a top level of enterprise systems fed by individual organizational systems.

Each of these approaches has both advantages and disadvantages, and none has yet emerged as the preferred technology approach for the IDS. Executives must realize that careful, rational evaluation of current capabilities aligned with future business vision will determine the best migration approach and path. Chapter Three deals with IT planning for integrated delivery systems in more detail.

Myth: Our vendor, systems integrator, application service provider, or outsourcer is our partner.

Reality: Final responsibility for information management must stay within the organization.

Cooperative, consultative relationships with vendors, systems integrators, application service providers (ASPs), and outsourcing organizations are important and offer significant benefits to health care organizations. However, these relationships cannot take the place of management competency in information technology decision making by executives within the health care organization. In addition, a health care organization that becomes too reliant on a vendor *or a vendor company's vision* can miss important technological shifts or advances developed elsewhere in the market.

In forming and maintaining effective relationships with these outside organizations, health care providers and payers must recognize the incentives driving these organizations. When discussing "at-risk" relationships, providers and payers should accept partnership status only when there is risk parity between the supplier and the organization.

Myth: Health care is underspending on information technology.

Reality: The situation is more complicated than it may seem.

It has long been accepted that compared to other knowledge- or service-based industries, health care underspends on IT. Gaining an accurate picture of reality is somewhat more complicated than simply stacking dollar volumes and percentages up against each other.

In any IT budget, a certain allocation will be spent in areas close to the heart of the organization, that is, core applications and technologies that support day-to-day transactions, operations, and communications requirements. In integrated delivery systems, this allocation represents the vast majority of IT budget dollars, which today is generally expected to be between 2.5 and 3.5 percent of the organizational operating budget.

What, then, accounts for the difference between IDSs and, say, banks, which typically spend 10 to 14 percent of their budgets on information technology? Banks invest significantly more money in *advanced* technology—data warehousing, data mining, customer service, and interactive marketing technologies that help them remain competitive. For example, in the banking industry, there are beta sites up and running that use retinal scanning on automated teller machines in lieu of passwords. A bank spending 10 percent on IT may devote 4 percent to core transaction systems, 4 percent to marketing and customer retention systems, and 2 percent to strategic and decision support technologies.

Health care, as an industry, has historically devoted the bulk of its IT dollars to the first area, core transaction systems, while spending far less in or completely ignoring the other areas. So in one sense, health care does spend competitively with other industries. Where the health care industry falls behind is in technologies that can create and sustain advanced market competencies. Today, new technologies with wide reach and maneuverability (such as the Internet) offer the opportunity to match other industries' system models, allowing for investments in advanced technologies without prohibitive costs.

What is important is not an IT dollar-for-dollar comparison between unrelated industries but rather the timely investment in technologies that offer sufficient benefit in health care: improvements in cost, service, and clinical outcomes.

Myth: New systems replace old systems.

Reality: Nothing replaces anything.

It is extraordinarily rare for a rational planning and information technology development approach to support a complete start-over. In today's health care marketplace, an overwhelming number of organizations expand their IT investments incrementally. Certainly, direct replacements (such as a new pharmacy system or a new financial system) frequently occur, but in general terms, the IT infrastructure at health care provider and payer organizations does nothing but grow over time.

There are a number of IT management implications to this growth pattern. IT departments must do all of the following:

- Be capable of supporting an increasingly diverse portfolio of applications, targeted at a broad group of end users (administrative management, clinical staff, financial analysts, and so on)

- Make available a broad range of data and information access tools (computers, workstations, wireless, telephone, handheld) to meet the different needs of end user constituencies

- Take advantage of data integration and user-directed tools to provide cost-effective data access and transaction management across organizations and functions wherever possible

- Have staff capable of handling the support requirements of both the number of diverse technology applications and the number of end users

THE IMPORTANCE OF EXECUTIVE KNOWLEDGE

Each IT-related myth we have discussed underlines the need for information technology planning to focus consistently on the larger goals and requirements of the health care organization. Without a greater organizational focus to support, IT will be limited in its effectiveness and capabilities. Similarly, if the larger organization doesn't understand the fundamental capabilities made possible through information technology, the organization will be limited in its accomplishments.

For the health care executive, this translates into a requirement for a direct and continually updated knowledge base about the needs, capabilities, and possibilities of health care IT. Specific *technical* knowledge is not required per se, but rather a business view of what IT tools are available and how they might be applied to specific health care issues. A clear goal of this work is to give readers the tools they might need to develop and mature such a business perspective.

THE TECHNOLOGY OF HEALTH CARE

In-depth discussions of systems programming, computer operating systems, and hardware are beyond the scope of this book and beyond the needs of executive management. This guide focuses on the areas of health care IT about which health care executives must be informed if they are to manage effectively. Particular attention is paid to information technology that has a strong impact on business direction, medical service goals, and financial results.

The scope and focus of information technology in health care has broadened considerably since the days of "data processing" at the hospital. Today, *information technology* refers to any technology designed to facilitate process or customer service automation. In health care, IT encompasses application software, Internet and intranets, computer operating systems, database and data access systems, telecommunications, networking, and computer hardware.

Tables 1.1 and 1.2 present a general overview of the information systems and technology covered in this book; Chapter Two provides a more in-depth look at features and functions.

Health care application systems include software programs that are designed to support users (employees, clinicians and physicians, patients, enrollees) in their activities during the course of their daily work. Some of these systems support relatively defined tasks, such as claims processing and patient billing. Others give users the capability to conduct more complex or less defined tasks, as when clinical decision support systems use complicated algorithms to assist clinicians in direct patient care activities.

Health care foundation and advanced technologies include technologies that allow application systems to communicate more effectively (a data integration tool, integration of computer and telephone technology) or that have the potential to broaden the fundamental delivery reach of an application (Internet, electronic commerce).

Table 1.1. Health Care Application Systems

Application System	Overview Description
Clinical systems	These systems support the activities of clinicians providing direct patient care, including presentation of clinical data, clinical documentation, and workflow. Advanced clinical support tools such as alerts and pathways are sometimes included in this category of application.
Consumer and patient health systems	Focus and functionality vary, but these systems are universally targeted for direct use by health care consumers. Very commonly, these systems will offer some form of educational and data tracking and storage capabilities designed to help patients self-manage their medical or health experiences. Patient-interactive systems directly involve patients in the care experience, providing guidance in triaging health problems, access to appointment scheduling capabilities, ongoing disease or medication management regimens, and communication with care providers.
Core transaction systems	These systems provide the basic financial, administrative, and clinical functionality required to maintain current operations, including initiating, tracking, and billing for both inpatient and outpatient care. Systems are generally customized for location of care delivery and may include functions for hospitals, independent practice associations (IPAs), management services organizations (MSOs), physician offices, home health organizations, and long-term care facilities.

Table 1.1. Continued

Application System	Overview Description
Decision support systems	These systems provide advanced support for operational, financial, and clinical decision making, including analysis tools to make judgments about clinical care, lines of service, and financial management.
Electronic medical record	This technology aggregates patient data from a variety of source systems; advanced electronic medical records allow access to text, graphics, clinical results, images, voice, or video.
Enterprise systems	These systems allow single points of access for patient and resource management.
Managed care systems	Designed to support the extended requirements that managed care places on organizations, these systems offer advanced administrative, clinical, and financial capabilities. System functionality varies by the type of user organization (for example, provider or payer).
Medical management systems	Clinically oriented, these systems are designed to assess or guide clinicians in the process of care provision, playing a preemptive "quality control" role in the care process. By delivering and integrating clinical content such as clinical protocols, alerts, reminders, drug interaction and allergy information, and formularies across care locations, these systems help organizations manage care for optimum outcome at lowest cost.

Table 1.2. Health Care Foundation and Advanced Technologies

Technology	Overview Description
Clinical data repository or data warehouse	This technology provides storage for partial or complete sets of organizational data, both clinical and financial. May be used to provide immediate access to data or allow for longitudinal collection and analysis of patient population health data.
Computer-telephony integration	This technology combines the use of telecommunications technology with application systems. Most commonly used with call centers, nurse triage, and educational and consumer-oriented efforts.
Customer relationship management	Application systems utilizing computer-telephony integration to document, track, and manage customer contacts with the organization.
Data integration	This technology, often custom-programmed by a systems integrator, allows free connectivity between existing application systems. Through data integration, patient demographic data input at one point of care can be accessed and reused at any other. May also include "off the shelf" applications such as interface engines and data repositories.
Electronic commerce technology	Electronic commerce technology incorporates a combination of application system and advanced technology to allow consistent, secure, and reliable communication across often unconnected entities. Most developed in health care supply chain systems and claims, authorization, and eligibility transaction processing.
Imaging	Systems that support the collection, viewing, and manipulation of digital images, whether documents, patient pictures, or clinical results data.

Table 1.2. Continued

Technology	Overview Description
Integrated medical devices	These allow the capture, collection, and transmission of physiologically oriented patient data into health care application systems. An example of this technology would be a peak flow meter that allowed the periodic download of readings onto the physician's desktop.
Internet, intranet, and extranet connectivity	Rapidly becoming the major delivery mechanism for large data sets, this technology is central to pioneering efforts in organizational marketing and "branding," patient education and consumer health, internal workflow redesign, and cost reduction. Core transaction system vendors are almost universally exploring it as a technology platform for application functionality.
Research systems	Systems that allow the collection, consolidation, tracking, management, and analysis of data relating to clinical research efforts. They include administrative, financial, and clinical data components.
Telemedical and telehealth technologies	These allow for clinical diagnosis and treatment support across geographical distances. Systems support the bidirectional transmission of voice, text, and imaging data.
Workflow technologies	Often integrated into application systems, workflow technologies support the work processes of computer end users. Smart routing used by call center technologies or automated work queues for medical management staff would be included in this category.
Workforce-enabling technologies	Technologies that support the education and training of organization staff, as well as communication between them. They include technologies such as electronic mail, groupware, knowledge management tools, Internet and intranet access, computer-based continuing education, and distance learning.

TRENDS AFFECTING THE HEALTH CARE PROVIDER MARKET

The use and development of health care information technology is strongly influenced by business, health care, and technology trends. Important current trends include the maturation of the hospital segment, the transition to an enterprise care model, the expansion of the information society, and short-term regulatory and technology pressures.

Maturation of the Hospital Segment

Over the past decade, across the hospital industry, the basic level of understanding, comfort, and capability—or core competency—in information technology has been permanently elevated. In the United States, certain basic hospital transaction functions (such as patient accounting, patient registration, and laboratory test processing) are now nearly universally automated. The hospital segment has moved from a technology-neutral orientation to one of technological awareness and adoption. Other segments, such as physician group practices and long-term care, lag, sometimes considerably, behind.

Foundation and advanced technologies like the Internet and electronic commerce today allow for greater sophistication in communications *between* health care entities. However, creating effective links between organizations requires that both have a certain level of IT capability. Today, hospitals and mature IDSs are more capable than other health care organizations of creating and sustaining this link. Payers and outpatient, ambulatory, and ancillary care providers must focus on developing an infrastructure and competency in information technology.

Transition to an Enterprise Care Model

The health care industry is clearly focused on the evolving enterprise model of care, with two-thirds of all community hospitals reporting participation in either a health system or a health network.[1] Enterprise

---

[1] American Hospital Association, *Hospital Statistics* (Chicago: Health Forum, 2000, p. 8). Data for 1998.

technology solutions are no longer being viewed as purely an additional application suite; rather, many organizations are requiring these functions as part of the minimum specification set for a technology purchase.

As health care providers transition to this enterprise model, some of the planning and investment issues around information technology change. For one thing, as a single organization, a health system represents a larger point of purchase for an information technology vendor than a stand-alone hospital does. As such, the organization may wield significantly greater power and influence over the terms of an IT purchase. On an even larger scale, group purchasing programs and cooperatives, including University Healthsystem Consortium, VHA, and Premier Health Alliance, have proved this theory by developing "preferred" discounts for participating members.

In spite of this greater influence, most health systems are discovering that enterprise system implementation is an expensive proposition. The systems are complex and require broad resources and process overhaul to implement. Executives must evaluate whether the return from enterprise standardization of systems will actually provide sufficient financial impetus to justify these costs.

Developing an enterprise architecture that allows distributed data capture and access increases the importance of data security, data standards, data dictionaries, and data update and prioritization procedures. A single mistake in an enterprise environment can cascade into multiple databases, creating and magnifying disarray to multiple points of service.

Finally, "one-stop shopping" has yet to become a reality in enterprise models. To date, no vendor has proved capable of offering an enterprise-wide solution that meets every health system need. The difficulty of finding a single acceptable system, and the largely unachieved value of combining financial and clinical data in a single repository, has resulted in many health care organizations developing financial and clinical applications along separate pathways.

The Information Society

Today's health care organization is competing with other health care providers to capture, retain, and serve patients. Consumers are increasingly looking across service industries to evaluate and compare the capabilities of various organizations; health care, unfortunately, usually comes up short when compared in such a manner.

Today's consumer expects not only attentive service from organizations but also instant or near-instant access to information. In today's world, an individual can have his paycheck electronically allocated and routed to multiple personal bank accounts; use almost any ATM to check instant account balances, route loan payments, or get cash; buy and sell stocks on-line; order a pizza or fried chicken by providing his telephone number, which is enough information for the restaurant to pull up name, driving directions, and food and payment preferences; and maintain a personal or family health record on-line, receive medication reminders, order prescriptions and supplies, or search medical literature without the aid or consent of his usual health care provider.

Yet the same person, during the course of obtaining and paying for health care, must often fill out redundant forms and make multiple phone calls to schedule services, talk to a care provider, complete payment, and resolve questions.

Partly in response to new activism among consumers, many organizations have begun to explore consumer-oriented health care information systems. Many of these systems have focused on educational, specific disease management, and individual data tracking capabilities, but some organizations are implementing Internet, intranet, and extranet and interactive voice response systems that allow appointment scheduling, prescription refills, and direct provider communication capabilities.

Short-Term Technology and Regulatory Pressures

For some time now, short-term technology and regulatory pressures have presented formidable planning and implementation challenges to health care provider and payer organizations.

For one thing, compliance requirements for the Health Insurance Portability and Accountability Act (HIPAA) are moving to the front of organizational radar. The electronic data standards requirements of the act will prove difficult enough for many providers and payers to come into compliance with; more challenging to implement, however, may be the data tracking and management demands of the confidentiality provisions of the legislation.

Furthermore, continued oversight pressure and concern about Medicare fraud and compliance have caused many organizations to devote specific intense resources toward IT-related evaluation and prevention mechanisms.

While these immediate pressures often capture the lion's share of executive focus and attention, organizations that allow them to distract from other medium- and long-term priorities *do so at their own risk*. Managed care changes, price and cost pressures, mergers and acquisitions, and state and federal regulations all contribute to short-term turbulence, but executives can successfully navigate the waters by planning on multiple planes, both proactively and reactively to market requirements.

THE HEALTH CARE IT MARKET: SUPPLIER SEGMENTS

Health care organizations continue to rely heavily on commercial application software and hardware vendors as well as systems integrators to supply required information technology. Like the provider and payer markets, the technology supplier market has undergone considerable turbulence and evolution.

The quality, timeliness, and effectiveness of the information technology developed and sold by supplier or vendor companies are affected by the shape of the current market as well as business, health care, and technology trends.

Information technology suppliers can be divided into five subgroups. Each subgroup offers a range of systems and services that are targeted to different types of organizations as well as buyers within organizations. The five subgroups are as follows:

1. *Health care application software and service providers.* These vendors typically offer products that automate a user's business and information needs. Solutions may be comprehensive or geared to one or more specialized areas. Companies operating in this market segment vary according to the business function served. Examples include hospital, physician, home health, payer and health plan, laboratory, pharmacy, nursing, and decision support application submarkets.

2. *Internet-intranet-extranet software and service providers.* This is the newest vendor market serving health care providers and payers. These vendors are attempting to build from the competencies of *all other information technology submarkets* to create added-value application functionality served over the Internet or over a private organizational intranet or extranet. They may directly target consumers, employers, or provider or payer organizations with their offerings and services.

3. *Original equipment (hardware) manufacturers.* These vendors provide the equipment that runs the application software, as well as peripheral devices such as printers, personal computers, and computer terminals.

4. *Telecommunications and network services suppliers.* These systems connect various peripheral devices, organizations, and enterprise sites via computer and telephone networks. These vendors are rapidly gaining in prominence as provider organizations become more geographically decentralized. This group includes Internet service providers (ISPs), the organizations that actually provide access to the Internet.

5. *Consulting services, systems integration companies, and outsourcing firms.* These labor and material suppliers offer business and technology planning, process reengineering, technical and functional systems integration services, and operations and management outsourcing capabilities. They are ideal for providers and payers struggling with connectivity between numerous legacy systems and new technologies or for organizations embarking on significant self-development efforts. They may also provide excellent support to organizations experiencing rapid transition, burgeoning IT cost structures, or extremely poor customer satisfaction.

Table 1.3 identifies the basic features and characteristics of each of these submarkets.

Table 1.3. Comparison of Information Technology Market Providers

Type of Supplier	Market Focus	Characteristics	Examples
Health care application software and services	Sale, installation, and maintenance of transaction and other application systems identified in Table 1.1.	Core group of companies with install base of client sites; upcoming group with newer technologies gaining ground; "one-hit wonders" with up to five beta sites that never go anywhere.	Cerner Epic Systems Corporation IDX McKesson/HBOC Medicalogic Meditech Siemens/SMS Sunquest
Internet-intranet-extranet software and services	Developing and marketing systems that rely solely on Internet or intranet delivery platforms; a subset of the larger application market. *Provider-based* companies focus on developing and selling solutions to providers and payers. *Consumer-based* companies focus on applications appealing to individuals, patients, and citizens.	Rely heavily on characteristics, technologies, and competencies from all other market segments.	Drugstore.com (consumer) Eclipsys (provider) Gaiam.com (consumer) HealthVision (provider) Medibuy.com (provider) Quadramed (provider) Vitacost.com (consumer) WebMD (both provider and consumer) Wellmed.com (consumer) *(Table continued on next page)*

Table 1.3. Continued

Type of Supplier	Market Focus	Characteristics	Examples
Original equipment (hardware)	Provide equipment used to operate application software; office automation systems; database tools and report writers.	Core providers extremely dominant; strongly affected by move to open systems and declining cost of PC ownership; close links to application software market vendors.	Compaq Dell Hewlett-Packard IBM SUN
Telecom and network services	Local and wide area networking technology; telephone connectivity, PBX systems; Internet service providers.	May or may not provide equipment; rapidly expanding market; historically less centered around the health care market.	AT&T Cabletron Systems Cisco Systems Interland Lucent Technologies Nortel Networks Synoptics 3Com

Table 1.3. Continued

Type of Supplier	Market Focus	Characteristics	Examples
Consultants, systems integrators, and out-sourcers	Advisory or direct technical expertise in systems issues, including planning, vendor selection, systems devel-opment, implementation, connectivity, and out-sourcing.	Service capabilities may or may not be health care centered.	Accenture CSC EDS Ernst & Young First Consulting Group Information Technology Optimizers Perot Systems SAIC Superior Consulting Trizetto Group

TRENDS AFFECTING THE SUPPLIER MARKET

The health care IT supplier market will face some unique challenges over the next few years. The *provider* world's continued transition to enterprise care models is forcing technology suppliers to reexamine their own business and development models, effecting a transition of their own, shifting from a stand-alone, feature-and-function approach to an enterprise-oriented, data sharing and exchange view.

Three of the current trends affecting this market are the crowding of the playing field, the uncertainties of the public investment market, and the evolution toward value-centered services.

The Crowded Playing Field

With more than three thousand firms offering application software or related services to the industry, the IT supplier market is both crowded and diverse. Despite the number of participants, revenues for the industry are concentrated in a very small number of active companies. One Top 100 list of health care IT firms for 1999 showed aggregate revenues of nearly $14 billion, with the largest ten firms accounting for more than one-half of that total.[2]

Fundamentally, the health care industry is struggling to provide more seamless communications, services, and processes to its consumer base, using a far-flung and sometimes wildly divergent pool of technologies and application systems. For technology suppliers, this sets up a competitive market with staggered levels of competition—several "eight-hundred-pound gorillas" trailed by a larger pool of established $20 million firms, followed by an even larger class of emerging and embryonic organizations.

Health care organizations must reasonably plan for some amount of turbulence in their vendor relationships as companies merge or are acquired and as product lines are developed, expanded, ported to new technology platforms, or discontinued.

---

[2]"Healthcare Informatics 100," *Healthcare Informatics,* 2000, *17,* 55–102.

The Public Investment Market

For a number of years, the United States investment markets were extraordinarily good to the health care information technology (HCIT) industry. A lucrative bull market, growing revenues, and a driving need for capital funding pushed both the public and the private capital markets into the health care IT sector. HCIT firms have directly and indirectly benefited from this capital influx. Companies have gone public, and public companies have acquired other firms to meet or fuel earnings and revenue expectations. In recent times, however, earnings expectations, business failures, and tightening access to funds have placed serious pressure on HCIT firms of all sizes.

This pressure has felled more than one executive and company, generating corporate rebuilding efforts, customer and shareholder lawsuits, and in some cases, jail terms. Some health care organizations have taken advantage of this market, through development site revenue sharing or equity partnerships with technology suppliers who later go public. All of a supplier's customers benefit from well-spent cash infusions, which might go to fund further product development or transition to new technology platforms.

The Evolution Toward Value-Centered Services

As the hospital market segment becomes more universally automated, vendors selling hospital-oriented systems begin competing in a *replacement market* and must adjust their strategy as new sales become more difficult and become subject to pricing and competitive pressures. To maintain and grow their business, technology suppliers have several options:

1. Reduce price or increase service in an effort to compete effectively

2. Diversify their product line, selling additional systems to existing clients

3. Diversify their market space, selling systems in new market segments

Many information technology suppliers have reacted to the changing market by blurring the line between application *software* (providing a tangible product) and application *services* (providing a service supporting or supported by a product). Numerous application software firms (including

McKesson/HBOC and Siemens/SMS) provide facilities, outsourcing, or interim management services in addition to products. Others (including e-commerce-oriented firms like WebMD and ProxyMed) are attempting to translate their service-based competencies into successful application software, consumer, and e-commerce markets.

For the application systems vendor, this trend means developing new ways to add value to old offerings. Firms like Cerner Corporation and CSC have purchased or developed entire consulting divisions around their deep proprietary product and integration knowledge. For the traditional application services vendor, it means developing competency in tangible product development, sales, and ongoing support. The transition for these firms seems to be more difficult, with few notable success stories.

What does this mean for health care providers and payers? It is essential to evaluate the company behind each product and service, examining its business direction, core and advanced competencies, and strategic alliances *in addition to the product or service being considered.* A vendor's product or service should fit the organization's vision, *not* vice versa. In a situation where the reverse is true, where an organization must wrap its vision around a service or product, the "fit" between the organization and the service or technology is not good, and a sudden shift by the supplier into a new, incompatible market would increase the provider organization's vulnerability.

Other important considerations should include the technology company's financial status, its demonstrated commitment to future product development, the reputation of executive leadership within the firm, the existence of a clearly articulated corporate vision, and the organization's customer support model and track record on client satisfaction.

SUMMARY

The development and application of information technology in health care has changed tremendously over the past decade and continues to evolve in ways that offer extraordinary potential for the delivery and management of health care. The nature of technology, technology vendors, and the trends affecting the marketplace all affect the utility of health care information technology. To take full advantage of this potential, CEOs and other executives must understand the market as well as the capabilities of IT and competently apply technology-focused management to their core business: delivering health care and improving the health of their patient populations.

CHAPTER 2

Information Systems Features and Functions

Like the provider and payer organizations they serve, health care information technology vendors have been evolving from a discrete point-of-service focus toward a continuum of care support. Departmentally focused systems that don't accept and exchange data with other applications are slowly disappearing, as HCIT suppliers develop and extend data exchange capabilities and health care organizations pour money into application integration.

Today, an amazing breadth and variety of applications are available, on "traditional" as well as Internet-based delivery platforms. Understanding the multidimensional power of these systems requires more than a simple discussion of core features. As the health care architecture expands to include intranet, extranet, and Internet capabilities, organizations must now decide not only which technologies and applications to implement but also *at what point* in the architectural continuum to apply them.

Return on investment (ROI), a long-standing industry challenge, assumes greater importance in the new (Internet-intranet-extranet) model of technology management. The added complexity of systems planning and implementation makes feature and function analysis, benefits projection, quantification, and architectural planning critical long-term success factors. Health care organizations are taking a variety of approaches to measuring

ROI, each aimed at establishing an appropriate mixture of technologies, applications, features, and functions.

THE NEW HEALTH CARE ARCHITECTURE

The traditional architecture has offered organizations a one-dimensional view of systems, with function and use focused primarily on users from within a single organization. Today's environment requires considerably more systems intricacy, with advanced financial and clinical applications supported by foundation technologies. These systems and technologies enable organizations to reach an increasingly diverse body of users, establishing and maintaining communications pathways both within and outside the organization.

The Foundation Technologies

Foundation technologies are enablers, rather than straightforward application systems. Some, like the Internet and computer telephony or interactive voice response, are delivery platforms that extend the overall reach of the health care organization. Others, like workflow systems and integrated medical devices, fundamentally change the nature of one or more organizational processes.

Foundation technologies include the following:

- *Internet-intranet-extranet:* Large public or private networks allowing for broad connectivity and access to data and systems
- *Data repositories or warehouses:* Technology storing large or extremely large data sets, particularly of clinical or financial data
- *Data integration tools:* Systems or technologies allowing the connection of disparate systems through data mapping or translation capabilities
- *Computer telephony and interactive voice response:* The integration of computer and telecommunications technologies to allow for directed use of telephones
- *Electronic commerce (e-commerce):* The electronic exchange of data, goods, or services for financial remuneration (also electronic)

- *Integrated medical devices:* Technologies allowing the capture, collection, and transmission of physiologically oriented patient data into health care application systems

- *Workflow systems:* Application systems that support work processes of end users, through "smart" routing or automated work queues

- *Imaging systems:* Systems that support the collection, viewing, and manipulation of digital images, whether document-based or radiological

While each of these technologies has played and continues to play an important role in health care information technology, the Internet has had the most revolutionizing effect on HCIT development, planning, and implementation.

The Internet as Change Driver

Efforts to integrate health care—community health information networks, vertically and horizontally integrated delivery systems, disease management programs, multidisciplinary care planning, and case management—have all been partly successful in broadening the view of care delivery. None of these models, however, has been able to offer the reach, infrastructure, or acceptance necessary to motivate wide-scale change.

The Internet may well offer all three.

Now that nearly one-half of the country's population has access to the Internet, that medium is exceeded in reach only by basic communications channels such as telephone, television, and radio. Today's Internet consumer can book airline flights, purchase just about anything, take virtual classes, even prequalify for home and car loans on-line.

The sheer volume of dollars spent on health care in this country make it an attractive marketplace for suppliers of products and services. Thanks to low market entry costs, Internet companies have flooded into the industry in an astonishing array of forms—e-doctors, e–health insurance companies, e-retailers, e-pharmacists, e-content portals, and others. Each offers consumers benefits in terms of added access, convenience, cost savings, or services.

So a health care organization's failure to maintain a Web presence or Internet-accessible services is more and more apparent to the public. Early adopters are already offering Internet- and extranet-enabled services to their patients, including secure messaging with providers, access to on-line appointment scheduling, and even maintenance of personal health records.

Adding "Net" Layers

These systems are made possible through the use of Internet and related technologies. Effective planning and implementation require organizations to adopt a layered system view, defining, at each layer, what features and functions to make available to which constituents.

Each layer can broaden access to a new group of constituents or offer old ones value over and above that already received. Figure 2.1 provides a brief summary of the Internet-intranet-extranet systems architecture.

A basic health care delivery function, patient registration, might assume a slightly different look at each layer of the architecture:

1. At the *core systems* layer, staff at each point of care are able to register patients as they present for appointments.

2. At the *intranet* layer, central staff can register patients for care at multiple locations, allowing patients with multiple appointments the convenience of a single point of access.

3. At the *extranet* layer, patients are allowed secure access to the organizational registration system, preregistering themselves for care. The information provided by the patient populates the core system, becoming immediately accessible by providers at the point of care.

The value offered, and the constituency most affected, changes at each layer, as the reach of the Internet is more fully integrated with the capabilities of the core systems layer.

The CEO's Guide to Health Care Information Systems

Figure 2.1. Internet-Intranet-Extranet Systems Architecture

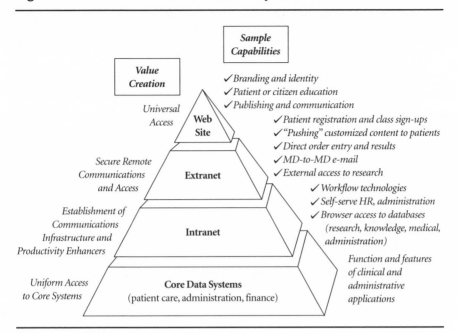

HEALTH CARE APPLICATION SYSTEMS

The breadth of available health care applications is staggering, with systems designed to meet administrative, financial, and clinical needs at any point of care. Throughout this chapter's discussion of functionality and return on investment, overlap across system "types" is included in the broadest possible sense—thus a discussion about physician profiling as an application system feature is included under both clinical decision support and medical management. For each application area, the impact of the Internet, including the functions most commonly Internet-based or -enabled, is also considered.

Core Transaction Systems

Core transaction systems provide the basic financial and administrative functionality for health care organizations to maintain their daily operations. As such, these systems typically touch all patient and organizational data in some way. They are used in all kinds of health care organizations, including hospitals, physician offices, long-term care facilities, home health organizations, and ambulatory surgery centers.

Individual applications falling within this category include the following:

- Patient administration and management
- General financial management
- Physician practice management
- Home health care management

As the central collection point for patient as well as organizational administrative and financial data, these systems are the most fully developed and most broadly implemented health care information systems.

Systems Overview. Patient administration and management systems (see Table 2.1) focus on the logistical requirements of organizations in preparing for patient care, tracking patients during care, billing and being reimbursed for care, and retrospectively evaluating care. (*Medical records systems,* sometimes considered part of this category, are discussed in a later section.)

General financial management systems (see Table 2.2) focus on the fiduciary responsibilities of health care organizations, including those to communities, employees, and external trading partners.

In smaller or less developed markets, core transaction systems and clinical systems are often sold as components of a single product. For example, in the physician practice and home health care markets, core transaction systems frequently offer some amount of clinical functionality.

Physician practice management systems (see Table 2.3) offer administrative, financial, and clinical functionality for independent physicians or group practices.

Table 2.1. Patient Administration and Management Systems

Function	Description
Admission, discharge, transfer	Handles the administrative requirements relating to initiating or ending care or moving an inpatient from place to place
Collections	Tracks and manages financial management for delinquent patient and payer accounts
Patient billing, accounts receivable	Assembles and monitors the claims submission and reimbursement process
Registration	Handles the administrative requirements of initiating or completing care or moving an outpatient from place to place
Scheduling (patient)	Incorporates patients, providers, rooms, equipment, other resources
Utilization review, quality assurance	Tracks appropriateness of care and reviews cases that deviate from quality or care standards

Home health systems (see Table 2.4) offer administrative, financial, and clinical functionality to support the daily activities of home health care provider organizations. In these organizations, information technology must be able to support the needs of the overwhelmingly mobile workforce. Foundation technologies such as wireless and electronic data interchange are commonly found integrated into these application systems.

Internet and E-Commerce Activity. One of the most common Internet and e-commerce functions relating to core transaction systems today is the

Table 2.2. General Financial Management Systems

Function	Description
Accounts payable	Tracks debts incurred by the organization; check writing
Budgeting	Manages budgets at the organizational as well as the departmental level
Fixed assets	Manages capital assets, including the depreciation process
General ledger	Handles general financial management and reporting
Human resources	Manages "human assets"—tracking and administration of benefits, staff assignments, education and training
Materials and equipment management	Orders and tracks supplies, miscellaneous equipment and maintenance
Payroll	Manages data collection, check writing, as well as tax withholding
Regulatory and tax reporting	Handles automated collection and assembly of required data
Scheduling (staff)	Schedules multidisciplinary staff in multiple locations with multiple methodologies
Time and attendance	Tracks employee work schedules and attendance

Table 2.3. Physician Practice Management Systems

Function	Description
Accounts receivable	Tracks receivables owed to organization for services provided; manages the claims submission process
General financial	Manages exchange of funds, expenses, payroll
Managed care	Supports basic managed care contract tracking and analysis; incorporates contract financial terms to support accurate claims generation and submission
Medical records	Documents physician-patient encounters including history and physical, diagnosis, and recommendations
Scheduling, registration	Coordinates patient visits with appropriate provider
Utilization review, case management	Ensures that patients receive high-quality, cost-effective care; tracks patient compliance

implementation and use of electronic mail, both for organizational staff and (less commonly) for registered inpatients. Another, for hospitals as well as a growing number of physician organizations, is a Web site, with some level of promotional material or interactive functionality. Allowing consumers access to basic information like facility directions, business hours, and contact information for particular departments has provided immediate payback to many organizations in increased customer satisfaction. More advanced organizations have found additional creative ways to use the Web:

• Offering "nursery cams" allowing geographically disparate families an immediate view of new family members

Table 2.4. Home Health Systems

Function	Description
Accounts receivable	Tracks receivables owed to the organization for provided services; manages multiple reimbursement plans and approaches and billing practices
Clinical documentation, pathways	Defines and documents general treatment protocols and interventions; tracks patient acuity levels, health status, and outcomes measures
General financial	Manages exchange of funds, expenses, and payroll
Human resources	Manages employee benefits, schedules employees appropriately according to their skills; provides mechanism for employees to track productive time
Managed care	Supports basic managed care contract tracking and analysis; incorporates contract financial terms to support accurate claims generation and submission
Materials management	Tracks inventory, orders and replenishes supplies; manages durable medical equipment
Patient management	Tracks patient insurance and eligibility for services, patient registration, and demographic information
Scheduling	Coordinates scheduling of multiple clinical resources according to defined care plan; optimizes geography and travel times between appointments

- Posting pretest regimens to improve patient awareness of testing requirements (for example, "Don't eat after . . ." or "Wear loose clothes")

- Allowing consumers or patients on-line access to appointment requests and appointment scheduling or preregistration, to reduce delays when patients call or present for care

Other first-generation Internet and e-commerce development in these areas has been focused predominantly on supply chain, claims management, and human resources. Some of the available functionalities include the following.

Supply Chain

- Electronic generation and management of purchase orders

- Integration with supply or inventory management to trigger purchase orders

- Electronic funds transfer between suppliers and the health care organization

- Vendor access to secure receivables status inquiries via health care organization extranet

Claims Management

- Electronic claims submission with basic electronic validation checks (no missing data, gender flags, alphanumeric fields)

- Electronic eligibility inquiry for affiliated payer organizations

- Electronic referral submittal and management

- Electronic authorization requests and management

- Electronic claims submission integrated with internal organizational work queues routing claims or remittances needing manual intervention to the appropriate staff

Human Resources

- Direct payroll and 401(k) deposits

- Static access via organization intranet to corporate policies and procedures, employee directories, job listings, and other information

- Interactive access via organization Web site to interactive recruiting functions (on-line job bank, on-line résumé submission, electronic messaging between recruiters and candidates)

- Interactive access via organization intranet to employee benefits (including the ability to modify or request changes) and work schedules

Decision Support Systems

As health care has become increasingly automated, the data analysis tools available to users have become fairly sophisticated. Over the past decade, a body of applications—referred to as *decision support systems*—has emerged to support both operational and clinical decision-making processes.

Decision support systems (DSS) have gained broad acceptance in the hospital and payer marketplace. Other industry segments (physician practice, ancillary services) have been slower in adopting them, at least in part because these systems require an amount of external data not feasible to provide without significant core transaction system automation. Most decision support systems are either clinical or financial in focus, and they are frequently used in concert with one or more data repositories.

Systems Overview. Financial DSS are used primarily to examine care that has been delivered or to forecast the impact of cost or volume variables on future care. Individual applications are identified in Table 2.5. Clinical DSS components are listed in Table 2.6.

Internet and E-Commerce Activity. As DSS are somewhat specialized and targeted at a limited body of users (financial and clinical executive management), there has not been a tremendous amount of movement toward

The CEO's Guide to Health Care Information Systems

Table 2.5. Financial Decision Support Systems

Function	Description
Budgeting	Manages organizational, departmental, service line detail financial data
Case-mix analysis	Measures provider use of resources relative to severity of patient illness
Cost accounting	Allocates clearly identified cost detail for departments and service lines (per procedure, per diagnosis-related grouping, per ambulatory visit grouping)
Market and network analysis	Models physician, specialty, and facility needs; identifies market share and areas of unmet demand
Outcomes management (financial)	Tracks resource utilization (actual and expected) by severity of case
Productivity management	Measures labor hours, staffing, and labor costs
Reimbursement modeling and contract management	Supports if-then forecasts, volume sensitivities, compares actual to expected or projected revenues or expenses by facility, by service, by payer, by contract, and by patient group

redevelopment for an Internet platform. What has occurred, however, is the porting of decision support functionality into clinical application systems as the utility of such functions becomes clear. *Clinical expert systems,* designed to support physician decisions at the point of care, in particular have been incorporated into other Internet-enabled application areas (such as automated laboratory or pharmacy order entry systems and stand-alone medical management systems).

Table 2.6. Clinical Decision Support Systems

Function	Description
Clinical expert systems	Support clinicians in care delivery by providing prompts, management plans for critical and routine events, sequencing, rules, and so on
Clinical knowledge-based systems	Catalogue reference data; are oriented to support or supplement clinical practice; may include best practice reviews, on-line and off-line reference guides
Clinical process improvement	Offers rules-based processing alerts, diagnostic and treatment prompts
Critical paths and protocols	Guide approved or appropriate treatment methods for particular diagnoses or types of cases, variance tracking, and research support
Outcomes management (clinical)	Reconciles expected and actual patient health results by type and severity of case
Physician and provider profiling	Permits peer comparison of physicians, based on practice patterns, treatments, drug usage, diagnosis, and so on; allows evaluation of case mix, outcomes, utilization patterns across facilities, and case mix and severity

Clinical Systems

Today, clinical systems functionality has extended beyond the traditional laboratory-pharmacy-radiology group to include ancillary and role-based systems, such as nursing and order management. As a group, these systems support the needs of clinicians providing direct patient care.

Individual applications falling within this category include general clinical and medical management.

Systems Overview. *General clinical, ancillary, and specialty site systems* support the basic documentation, data access, and clinical care support requirements of role-based clinical staff. Applications in this category may include those listed in Table 2.7.

Medical management systems (see Table 2.8) are designed to assess or guide clinicians in the process of care provision. These advanced care systems deliver clinical contents such as clinical protocols, alerts, reminders, and drug interaction, allergy, and formulary data directly into the hands of providers.

Internet and E-Commerce Activity. Like core transaction systems, clinical systems have been an area of intense focus for Internet and e-commerce development. However, despite broad interest and considerable research and development investment by technology suppliers, health care organizations have remained hesitant to shift these applications to Internet or e-commerce platforms. A number of issues complicate the planning and implementation of Internet-enabled clinical systems, including privacy and security issues, a lack of consistent state and federal regulation, and inconsistent data standards within and across organizations.

Despite these barriers, technology adoption is occurring, with functions including the following:

- Electronic test orders and results reporting

- On-line consumer health status testing and measurement

- Electronic access to disease state information

- Electronic prescription orders and refills

- (*More advanced*) Secure integrated medical device readings (for example, peak flow for asthmatics, glucometer for diabetics) automatically uploaded and sent to clinical databases for review and possible intervention alerts

- (*More advanced*) Automated prescription refill notices, with alerts for possible patient noncompliance sent to ordering physicians

Table 2.7. General Clinical, Ancillary, and Specialty Site Systems

Function	Description
Nursing	Provides support for documentation requirements as well as workflow
Order management	Includes direct order entry as well as results reporting and display
Cardiology Emergency Laboratory Pharmacy Radiology Surgery	Supports the unique clinical and administrative needs of the various ancillary and specialty departments

Electronic Medical Record

We use the term *electronic medical records* (EMR) to refer to all forms of computer-based patient records, which may go by many names in the industry but strive for the same or very similar goals. EMR technology aggregates patient data from a variety of source systems, allowing access to text, graphics, clinical results, images, voices, or video. Development pathways for EMR technology have varied significantly, leading to a diverse marketplace that supports applications in a number of important areas.

Systems Overview. Applications in this category typically focus on administrative data-gathering requirements, clinical data documentation and storage, and clinical workflow support. Table 2.9 describes each area.

Not every EMR vendor addresses each of these functional areas with the same importance. A system designed for a hospital environment may have a sophisticated administrative medical records component, while a

Table 2.8. Medical Management Systems

Function	Description
Acuity	Measures or classifies the seriousness of illness or injury for a specified patient condition
Case management	Ensures that specific patients receive appropriate and cost-effective care
Disease management	Targets specific or "at risk" populations to permit better management of health care cost effectiveness and use
Outcomes	Generally focuses on clinically based measures and post-discharge tracking of patients
Physician or provider profiling	Focuses on practice patterns, treatments, drug usage, diagnosis, and the like, as well as on case mix, outcomes, utilization patterns across facilities, and severity of illness
Protocols	May be clinically derived protocols or simply treatment "pathways" with associated variance alerting and tracking
Utilization review, quality assurance	Tracks appropriateness of care and reviews cases that deviate from quality standards

physician office–centered system may place more emphasis on clinical documentation or workflow support capabilities.

Internet and E-Commerce Activity. Security and privacy are also core issues for technology developers porting EMR capabilities to an Internet platform. Internet and e-commerce development in this area has for the most part focused on secure remote access to data, with more advanced deployments incorporating workflow and messaging tools. Of note in this

Table 2.9. Electronic Medical Records

Function	Description
Administrative medical records	Include the administrative components of managing records; may include chart or deficiency tracking, abstracting and coding, and document imaging
Clinical data storage	Stores in a repository longitudinal patient data from multiple disparate points of care
Clinical documentation	Allows clinical users immediately to document or access clinical findings, progress notes, and other patient information
Clinical workflow support	Facilitates communication to and from providers, may organize work into role-based "queues"

area is the emergence of the consumer health record (also called a personal health record, or PHR), a patient-focused cousin to the EMR allowing for the collection and centralized storage of individual health information. (PHRs are discussed more fully in the section on consumer health systems.)

Internet and e-commerce functions developed in this area include the following:

- Static access to clinical data
- Drug interaction information
- Access to clinical protocols
- Consumer use of the PHR as a data repository
- Electronic routing and workflow prioritization of test results
- Secure messaging (provider-provider, provider-patient)

- Personal health record links to physician-based medical record
- Patient checks on status of insurance claims

Managed Care Systems

Managed care systems are designed to offer advanced administrative, clinical, and financial capabilities required for participation in managed care plans. Throughout the 1990s, the growth of managed care, especially the complexities inherent in capitated care arrangements, gave rise to this new set of functional requirements for provider and payer organizations.

At least in part due to the intensive cross-organizational data exchange required by managed care, electronic commerce has emerged as a dominant direction for these systems, notably including claims processing, eligibility, referral, and authorization activities.

Payer-based managed care systems continue to evolve and grow. On the provider side, however, many core transaction system vendors (particularly those at hospitals and physician practices) have incorporated these formerly specialized functions directly into their base systems. As such, a "stand-alone" provider managed care system has become increasingly rare and generally focuses on highly specialized activities (such as capitation and risk pool management or advanced contract analysis).

Systems Overview. Individual applications falling within this category are illustrated in Table 2.10. In addition to these, managed care systems may have separate modules for the administration of or participation in managed Medicare or Medicaid programs.

Internet and E-Commerce Activity. To some extent, the somewhat less well developed IT infrastructure at health care payer organizations has complicated the development and growth of Internet and e-commerce applications for these systems. Market interest is high; ability to execute, in most cases, is not, as payers struggle with decades of underinvestment in IT and custom-developed legacy applications.

Table 2.10. Managed Care Systems

Function	Description
Provider Managed Care Systems	
Claims	Formulates and submits claims
Contract management	Tracks actual versus expected (contracted) reimbursement; analyzes contract profitability
Eligibility, authorization	Collects and verifies patient eligibility and authorization requirements for service
Outcomes management	Tracks financial or clinical outcomes
Utilization review, case management	Monitors care usage and compliance with recommended care
Health Plan Managed Care Systems	
Capitation	Manages capitated contracts, including stop-loss and risk pool administration
Claims	Accepts and adjudicates claims; issues appropriate payments to providers
Contract management	Maintains provider fee schedules and contract terms; analyzes profitability by contract
Medical economics	Sets actuarial rates; performs advanced financial analysis
Member enrollment and eligibility	Collects administrative and clinical information necessary to manage patient experience, including contract and benefits coverage

Table 2.10. Continued

Function	Description
Member services	Tracks customer questions and concerns and assists in their resolution
Outcomes management	Tracks clinical or financial outcomes
Premium billing	Manages multiple group billing methodologies; performs individual billing for Medicare, COBRA, and other government agencies
Provider management	Tracks the credentials of participating physicians; performs physician profiling; matches authorization and referral data to claims
Utilization review, case management	Tracks and enters cases for precertification and concurrent review; handles discharge planning; matches services received with claims

The Health Insurance Portability and Accountability Act requires all plans to conform to electronic standards for claims, referral, eligibility, and authorization data. In preparation, a number of plans have already ported claims, eligibility, and authorization systems to Internet platforms, designing features and functions such as electronic claims submission and acceptance; electronic transmission of formulary, benefit plan, and participating physician data; and electronic transmission of eligibility and capitation rosters.

Enterprise Systems

Enterprise systems are application software programs that facilitate a single organizationwide point of access for a particular function, such as scheduling or materials management. A precursor to intranet- and extranet-enabled applications, enterprise systems began the IT industry shift toward broad and integrated access to data and system features.

Today, "enterprise" and "nonenterprise" systems are converging into a single set of applications designed to support organizations of large size and complexity. Though stand-alone systems still exist, many technology suppliers now offer a full suite of related, integrated applications (in such areas as materials management, purchasing, and human resources) or a basic application capable of expanding to meet the more complicated needs of larger delivery systems.

Systems Overview. The most common enterprise systems are shown in Table 2.11.

Internet and E-Commerce Activity. Internet and e-commerce development activity for these systems parallels those listed under their traditional counterparts.

Table 2.11. Enterprise Systems

Function	Description
Enterprise master patient index	Assigns and tracks unique identifiers for all patients entering the health care delivery system, irrespective of point of entry; links patient-related data resident in all systems through this identifier
Enterprise resource planning	Allows centralized management of materials, supply, and human resource functions, including purchasing, inventory, payroll, and regulatory reporting
Enterprise scheduling	Provides a single point of access to schedule caregivers, equipment, and rooms across the delivery system; uses scheduling logic to set up and sequence multiple appointments across multiple facilities

Consumer Health Systems

Historically, the health care industry has not equated the term *consumer* with *patient*, instead focusing on the economic consumer—typically an employer or a state or federal program subsidizing the cost of an individual's health care. The growth of the Internet, combined with increasing evidence of the benefits of population health management models, has fundamentally and permanently shifted the industry to a focus on the individual who actually receives health services.

Health care IT vendors have rushed to develop consumer health systems or applications that target services or functionality directly at the patient-consumer. While geared toward the individual as end user, most systems are designed for administration or funding through a health care organization—either a physician group, hospital, or health plan.

Systems Overview. Individual applications falling within this category are listed in Table 2.12.

The rapid availability of consumer-oriented health information has given rise to provider concern. No single entity holds legal or regulatory oversight responsibility for the incredible volume of health data now being offered to patients. Particularly in the case of the Internet, where medical- and pseudo-medical-related sites abound, "credentialing" content is a growing issue.

Internet and E-Commerce Activity. Currently the least developed of all application health areas, consumer health systems focus data exchange and electronic commerce capabilities on direct patient-provider communications and business-to-consumer electronic commerce. These systems are almost universally Internet- and e-commerce-focused, allowing for on-line (Web-based) data collection and capture and remote data storage and analysis, as well as e-commerce transactions such as prescription refills and retail purchasing.

Table 2.12. Consumer Health Systems

Function	Description
Disease and condition management	Coordinates record keeping and health management activities for conditions such as asthma, diabetes, headaches, congestive heart failure, pain, pregnancy, and pediatrics
Educational forums, "chat" groups, and similar	Focus on specific topic areas, including breast cancer, smoking cessation, weight loss, and depression
Health promotion	Allows users to coordinate individual health activities (such as fitness or nutrition) and planning
Health risk assessment	Presents standardized survey tools to measure health risks and wellness
Medical reference, education	Accesses proprietary and public health information at various levels of complexity
Messaging, e-mail	Enables patient-provider communication
Personal health record	Consumer version of the EMR; allows health record keeping
Retail health supplies	Accesses providers of health products and supplies, including on-line pharmacies and natural food stores

ADVANCED TECHNOLOGIES

In addition to the foundation technologies and application systems in widespread use today, there are any number of advanced technologies being developed, tested, and deployed at limited numbers of health care organizations (see Table 2.13). These systems typically offer highly specialized features or employ leading-edge technologies not widely available or adopted.

Table 2.13. Advanced Technologies

Function	Description
Biotechnology systems	Give bioinformatics companies and pharmaceutical firms the ability to manage data gathered in the efforts of gene sequencing, genomics, proteomics, and pharmacogenomics
Customer relationship management (CRM) systems	Use computer-telephony integration to manage contact and requests from customers; typically include call routing and logging, problem tracking, and resolution reporting
Research systems	Support the activities of clinical researchers, including grant tracking, physician-to-physician communications, research data tracking and analysis, proposal tracking, and electronic purchasing
Telemedicine and telehealth technologies	Support remote delivery of care; common features include image capture and transmission, voice and video conferencing, and text messaging
Workforce-enabling technologies	Include applications that provide computer-based training, video and voice conferencing, reference information and advanced search tools, document management, artificial intelligence, and intelligent transaction processing

SYSTEMS, TECHNOLOGY, AND RETURN ON INVESTMENT

It is important to remember that the end goal of any technology planning, evaluation, selection, or contracting process is not simply to obtain the technology. *It is to incorporate a particular technology's features and functions successfully into the daily operations of the organization, in the interest of fulfilling one or more specific organizational needs or requirements.*

Evaluating the features and functions of a technology or application system is an important part of meeting this goal, but not the only part. The possible benefits, and overall quantitative return on investment, should be examined in the context of current and future organizational business and medical service practices. ROI measurement has advanced considerably in recent years as more and more organizations have adopted quantitative measurement methods and approaches.

Fundamentally, however, ROI remains a function of management expectations, organizational risk tolerance, current systems and technology efficiency, organizational market position, and financial stability. Adopting an overall expectation for benefits and ROI (or a threshold that new investments must reach) is a critical first step to achieving value from information technology. Figure 2.2 describes a number of potential approaches to ROI.

Data Exchange and ROI

The most effective information technology framework is one in which, as much as possible, required data are passed between systems and across technologies with only as much human intervention as is truly required. Achieving that vision requires health care organizations to understand clearly the data interrelationships between systems.

Even a seemingly straightforward function like patient scheduling can become complex when you consider the actual data required to complete the task effectively (see Table 2.14). A scheduling system can potentially touch (either send data to or request information from) up to six other application systems. Accomplishing these exchanges effectively extends the utility and efficiency of any application system, correspondingly increasing return on investment.

Figure 2.2. Return-on-Investment Expectations

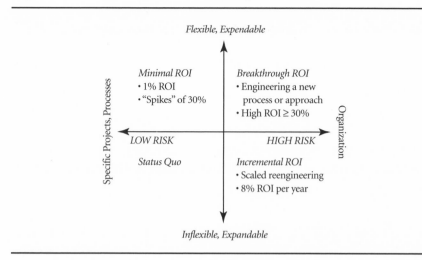

In approaching ROI measurement, organizations are taking a variety of both quantitative and qualitative approaches, including the following:

- *Best practices and benchmarking:* General review of ROI that other organizations have accomplished with the same technology; may include literature reviews or direct interviews with organizations.

- *Management engineering studies:* Detailed technical reviews of workflow, task effort and time requirements, and before-and-after reviews of technology impact.

- *Cost and feasibility analysis:* A mixed quantitative and best-practices approach, focusing detailed engineering and workflow analysis in critical areas or for higher-risk IT investments.

Irrespective of approach, any application system in use should support continued or increased capabilities by the health care organization staff. Some applications have clearly proved hard-dollar value; the financial benefits of electronic claims transmission and staff time and attendance systems, for example, have both been well documented. Other

Table 2.14. Patient Scheduling Data Exchanges

Originating System	Accepting System	Data Exchange
Patient administration	*Patient scheduling*	Verifies that patient exists in system
Patient administration	*Patient scheduling*	Communicates patient insurance, eligibility
Patient administration	*Patient scheduling*	Provides patient authorization and copayment requirements
Staff scheduling system	*Patient scheduling*	Verifies that staff required for appointment are available that day and time
Bed control or census	*Patient scheduling*	Verifies (inpatient) bed availability
Patient financial system	*Patient scheduling*	Checks for existing patient account balance
Patient scheduling	Dietary	Documents procedure-related dietary restrictions
Patient scheduling	Bed control or census	Provides notice to housekeeping to prepare
Patient scheduling	Medical records	Generates chart pull request
Patient scheduling	Patient financial system	Reconciles scheduled appointments with claims generated

systems have yet to prove their value, although the strategic advantages may be clear (these might include clinical workflow and messaging or clinical data repositories).

In each high-level IT investment area, the mixture of cash, efficiency, revenue, and strategic benefits returned will vary. Table 2.15 relates various typical returns for illustrated investments.

Benefit Mapping

Features and functionalities of technology are often mistaken for benefits. Many organizations place too much emphasis on selecting the broadest functional system without really considering what specific benefits the organization might attain from using the technology. It requires a conscious mapping process to turn features and functions into benefits.

In technology planning efforts, there are three methods to map the potential benefits of a specific application or technology. The first, moving from a defined business goal to a benefit, centers on the use of technology in supporting the clear business or medical service direction of an organization.

This approach does well when organizations have spent considerable time and effort defining their business and medical service objectives. However, it falls short in considering the strong impact health care IT can have in opening new business directions, particularly emerging technologies such as e-commerce and the Internet. The features and functions of these technologies can actually drive organizations to create new business goals.

Organizations that use both of these approaches may still face specific problems in operations. Under these circumstances, health care providers can often strategize to use technology in a way that mitigates (or resolves) the impact of the original business or medical service issue. Figure 2.3 shows how organizations can map business goals, technology potentials, or organizational problems into projected benefits.

Table 2.15. Investment Benefits

Technology Investment Areas:	Infrastructure	Core Transaction Systems	Enterprise and Emerging Technologies	Strategic and Decision Support	Information Systems Management
Examples:	Wide area network, databases, Internet	Practice management, laboratory and radiology, patient administration	Enterprise master patient index, enterprise resource planning, e-commerce, Internet-intranet-extranet	Clinical or population data repository	Outsourcing ASP model
Benefits					
Cash:	Low	First generation, high; second generation, medium; third generation, low	High	Medium	High
Efficiency (pivot point):	Medium	High	High	High	Medium
New revenues or earnings:	Low	Low	High	Medium	Low
Strategic positioning:	High	Low	High	High	Medium

Figure 2.3. Benefit Mapping

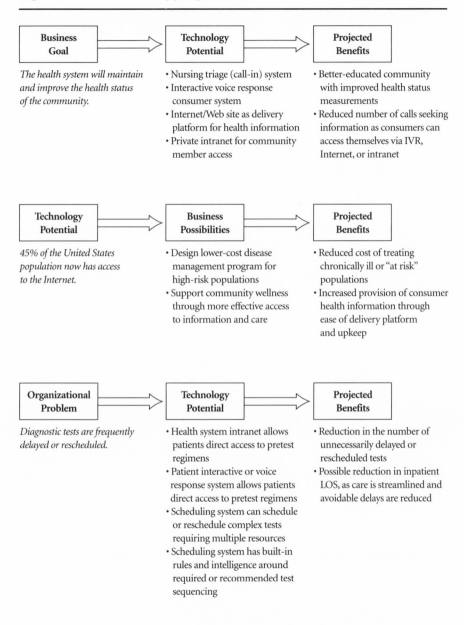

Business Goal	→	Technology Potential	→	Projected Benefits
The health system will maintain and improve the health status of the community.		• Nursing triage (call-in) system • Interactive voice response consumer system • Internet/Web site as delivery platform for health information • Private intranet for community member access		• Better-educated community with improved health status measurements • Reduced number of calls seeking information as consumers can access themselves via IVR, Internet, or intranet

Technology Potential	→	Business Possibilities	→	Projected Benefits
45% of the United States population now has access to the Internet.		• Design lower-cost disease management program for high-risk populations • Support community wellness through more effective access to information and care		• Reduced cost of treating chronically ill or "at risk" populations • Increased provision of consumer health information through ease of delivery platform and upkeep

Organizational Problem	→	Technology Potential	→	Projected Benefits
Diagnostic tests are frequently delayed or rescheduled.		• Health system intranet allows patients direct access to pretest regimens • Patient interactive or voice response system allows patients direct access to pretest regimens • Scheduling system can schedule or reschedule complex tests requiring multiple resources • Scheduling system has built-in rules and intelligence around required or recommended test sequencing		• Reduction in the number of unnecessarily delayed or rescheduled tests • Possible reduction in inpatient LOS, as care is streamlined and avoidable delays are reduced

SUMMARY

The development and application of information technology in health care has changed tremendously over the past decade and continues to evolve in ways that offer extraordinary potential for the delivery and management of health care. The nature of technology, technology vendors, and the trends affecting the marketplace all affect the utility of health care information technology. To take full advantage of this potential, CEOs and other executives must understand the capabilities of IT and judiciously apply technology-focused support to their core business: delivering health care and improving the health of their patient populations.

CHAPTER 3

The Integrated Delivery System

Over the past decade, historically separate health care industry submarkets (including hospitals, physician groups, long-term care providers, independent practice associations (IPAs), payers, and business coalitions) have come together in a new health care business model. This model, the *integrated delivery system* (IDS, sometimes called a *regional delivery system*), is designed to manage costs, apply a more even and complete continuum of care services, and preserve or increase revenues and market share.

Early adopters of this collaborative or combined delivery system model faced a complexity of business management, finance, physician integration, continuum of care, and information technology issues. Today, many of these early adopters have resolved and stabilized initial challenges and are moving on to face the far more complex questions relating to intra-IDS communication, technology and infrastructure, population health management, and large-scale data management and analysis. For other organizations, the road to integration still lies ahead.

There are multiple IDS care and business models operating in today's market; each offers key technological differences, advantages, and challenges. Whatever the approach or developmental stage, the nature of integration elevates strategic and tactical issues to a level of far greater complexity than those faced by stand-alone facilities.

DEFINING "INTEGRATED"

The reigning champion of buzz phrases in an industry infamous for them, *integrated delivery system* has come to symbolize all of the good, efficient, idealized structures and processes that health care *should* be. An integrated delivery system is coordinated and efficient with both medical care and the voluminous administrative data collection and management requirements of health care. In an IDS:

- Facilities provide consistent and high-quality care to their communities, with services geared to the specific needs and health status of their populations.

- Doctors can easily access patient histories and records, including data generated by and stored with other care providers and locations.

- Patients can provide required information at a single location, which then makes it accessible to all other associated providers and locations.

- Medical providers generate clear and understandable bills for services; charges are accurate and reasonable.

- Organizations combine financial and reimbursement integration with care planning, resulting in optimal care efficiency.

Organizations calling themselves "integrated" come in a wide variety of size, complexity, and structure, including business, operational, legal, financial, and information systems technology capabilities and strategies. Though few observers would deny that IDSs share the common goals of controlling costs, improving and maintaining care quality, and preserving or.expanding market share, considerable diversity in approach has emerged across the country.

The Components of Integration

There are a number of widely accepted characteristics of an integrated delivery system. It is important to note that not every IDS will have every component; each will, however, have at least some combination of the physical entities and medical and care structures listed in Exhibit 3.1.

Exhibit 3.1. Components of Integration

Physical Entities

- Regional or larger geographical scope

- Multiple acute inpatient facilities

- Freestanding and medical center–based ambulatory care

- One or more affiliated physician groups: may be owned (physicians are employees) or contracted for some amount of services

- Intermediate or long-term care organizations (such as skilled nursing or home health facilities)

- Home health and visiting nurse agencies

- Health plan capabilities (such as independent practice associations, management services organizations, third-party administrators, or fully licensed health plans)

- Managed care contracting organization

Medical and Care Structure

- Support for care components across the continuum, from inpatient acute to intermediate, long-term, and outpatient care

- Incorporation of physician organizations into the enterprise care model

- Focus on the management of patient populations

- Financial incentives ranging from case management incentives to some capitation and shared risk to full risk sharing

- Care integration

- "Center of excellence" focus

Central to the concept of an IDS is a focus on the continuum of care and continuity of care management. Where a particular organization may not offer a service line (say, long-term care), to be a "true" IDS, that organization must make that service available through an affiliation or a subcontract with another organization. *The key relationship with the patient remains heavily influenced (if not controlled) by the IDS structure.*

Fitting the Pieces Together

The "integrated" in *integrated delivery system* also implies some level of administrative and medical management coordination as a core feature of the organization. In fact, an IDS offers a complex mix of integrated components, touching on organizational structure, business strategy, care delivery, care financing, and information technology use.

Many organizations adopt a mixture of approach and intensity in each of these critical areas. (As the IDS evolves and strengthens, strategies and structures may change as well.) Table 3.1 identifies these areas and notes some key questions and decisions applying to each. The decisions made in each of these areas will significantly affect IT use and planning.

From Stand-Alone to Integration: General IT View

The focus of technology at the IDS level broadens considerably from stand-alone facilities. A uniform data and communications infrastructure (wide area network or intranet, universal system access and telecommunications) is an essential foundation for basic and advanced clinical and financial applications inherent in care integration. Equally of interest to the IDS is a uniform data view and single sign-on access for users, particularly clinical and administrative systems used by a broad audience.

Table 3.2 reviews IDS focus and critical applications.

MODELS OF INTEGRATION: COMMON APPROACHES

Although there is considerable variation in IDS structure and strategy, organizations tend to adopt one of four approaches: affiliation, regional delivery, affiliation with central services, or corporate ownership. Each approach reflects a range of ownership, operational and strategic vision, financial incentives, and information technology strategies.

Affiliation

In this model, organizations are loosely connected, driven to cooperate by interest in specific endeavors of mutual benefit (for example, large capital projects, disease management collaboration, specialty services, managed

Table 3.1. Five Integration Areas

Area	Questions and Decisions
Management	• Will the IDS have a centralized management function, or will individual entities be allowed their own governance structure? • How much control and latitude in making decisions will individual entities be allowed?
Financial	• Will balance sheets and assets be combined? • Will entities contract from a central function or individually? • How will risk be shared across entities?
Physician	• How large will the physician network be (primary care as well as specialty)? • Should practices be purchased or affiliated?
Continuum of care	• In developing a continuum of care, which service lines will be owned, which subcontracted, and which affiliated? • What degree of coordination will occur in care management efforts along the continuum? • For what diseases will structured management programs be put into place?
Information technology	• Will management and strategic planning be centralized, distributed, or both in combination? • What actual level of common systems will be required? • Will system architectures and approaches be mandated? Will a single vendor, best of breed, or cluster strategy be pursued?

Table 3.2. Key IDS Applications and Focus

System Type	IDS Focus	Critical IDS Applications
Core transaction systems	Enterprisewide view; data accessible via wide area network or intranet across IDS; possibly uniform systems; support central business operations as required	• Enterprise systems, including scheduling, master patient index, eligibility capabilities • Centralized payroll • Centralized materials operations • Financial management • Treasury functions
Decision support	Support of multiple organizations, entities, and service lines; applied to cost reduction, managed care contracting, clinical utilization and protocols	• Contracting and profitability analyses • Clinical case management, practice patterns • Actuarial or risk-adjusted outcome analysis • Patient or enrollee satisfaction • Budgeting (flexible and functional) • Productivity management
Clinical systems	Managing efficacy of care within contract or premium dollars allocated; must support entire continuum of care	• Common procedure, order protocols • Computerized protocols • Regional case, disease management solutions • Integrated ambulatory, acute care, and physician office results reporting

Table 3.2. Continued

System Type	IDS Focus	Critical IDS Applications
Electronic medical records	Single enterprise record; encounter-based longitudinal focus on patient or enrollee; aggregated data from multiple sources, uniform access	• Clinical data repository • Evolution away from purely administrative medical records toward clinical documentation and workflow support tools
Managed care systems	Contracting support; IDS structure frequently requires health plan functionality	• Contract management in support of multiple contracts • Capitation support • Health plan and third-party administrative systems
Foundation technologies	Support of geographical diversity; standardized backbone for reduced communications costs; integrated use of voice systems, fax capabilities, paging, and Internet and related network technologies	• Enterprise network or intranet standard sign-on and access • E-mail • Universal workstation • Clinical or financial data repositories • Workflow support tools • Imaging • Four-digit provider and patient dialing

(*Table continued on next page*)

Table 3.2. Continued

System Type	IDS Focus	Critical IDS Applications
Consumer health systems	Support for administrative, financial, and clinical needs	• Patient inquiry and self-service (appointment requests, account balance inquiry) • Personal health records and health risk assessment • Access to general and condition-specific health content data
Advanced technologies	Pilot implementations of relevant systems and technologies to support larger IDS goals	• Clinical research • Knowledge-sharing systems • Telemedicine, telehealth • Customer relationship management

care contracting). Organizations selecting this approach to IDS formation are commonly linked through a contractual or joint-venture relationship, as depicted in Figure 3.1.

The affiliation model is a very common "jumping off" point to move into an IDS strategy, allowing organizations to commit limited, focused resources to capture immediate or short-term benefits. This approach does not require participants to face the difficulties inherent in combining financial, management, and IT operations.

Figure 3.1. Affiliation IDS Model

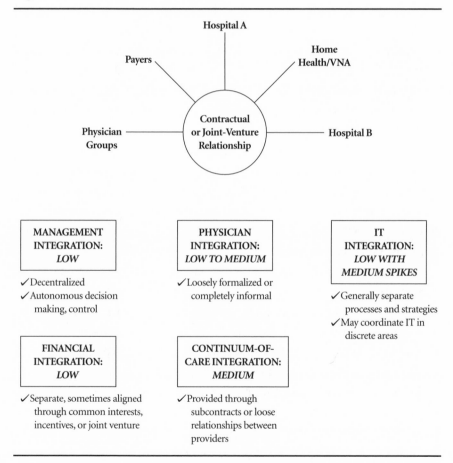

This model generally approaches information technology initiatives in the same fashion as other projects, judging on a case-by-case basis the need and advisability of jointly executing IT initiatives. Currently, the most common technology collaborations involve data sharing between entities. (One example might be the joint development of an eligibility or authorization lookup function allowing affiliated physicians to query payer databases about presenting patients. Another might be the sharing of specific cost, volume, and case data to support collaborative contracting efforts.)

Regional Delivery

Regional delivery is a recently emerged approach to IDS strategy and formation. For these organizations, integration is clearly a focus, while geographical reach is not. This model IDS typically works to develop a vertical continuum of services (for example, outpatient to inpatient to long-term care), often focusing on one to three "center of excellence" service lines, rather than a breadth of horizontal ones. Single hospital organizations are quite common, as depicted in Figure 3.2.

The regional delivery model is frequently adopted by organizations as a market preservation strategy, enabling them to control patient flow both into and outside the hospital. With more centralized management control than the affiliation model, the regional delivery model is well positioned to achieve greater levels of integration in financial, physician, care continuum, and information technology.

IT planning for the regional delivery model is similar to the corporate IDS approach, with at least a moderate level of centralization and control. Although a breadth of systems are required to support the continuum-of-care services, regional IDSs generally do not require a depth of systems (for example, to support multiple hospitals) or technological capabilities to reach as wide a geographical range. Applications and initiatives of particular focus for this model include centralized data repositories, enterprisewide clinical decision support systems, and Internet-intranet-extranet technology allowing affiliated physicians, organizations, and patients access to limited hospital-based and population and disease management health data.

Figure 3.2. Regional Delivery IDS Model

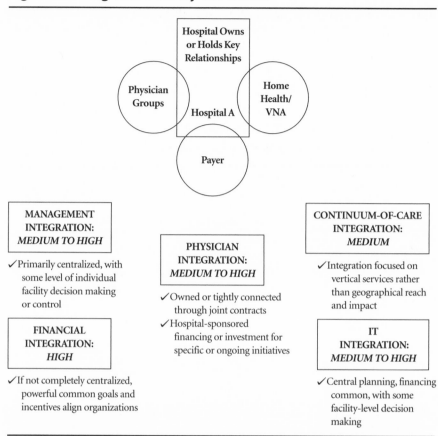

MANAGEMENT INTEGRATION:
MEDIUM TO HIGH

✓ Primarily centralized, with some level of individual facility decision making or control

FINANCIAL INTEGRATION:
HIGH

✓ If not completely centralized, powerful common goals and incentives align organizations

PHYSICIAN INTEGRATION:
MEDIUM TO HIGH

✓ Owned or tightly connected through joint contracts
✓ Hospital-sponsored financing or investment for specific or ongoing initiatives

CONTINUUM-OF-CARE INTEGRATION:
MEDIUM

✓ Integration focused on vertical services rather than geographical reach and impact

IT INTEGRATION:
MEDIUM TO HIGH

✓ Central planning, financing common, with some facility-level decision making

Affiliation with Central Services

Going a step beyond the affiliation approach, organizations affiliated with central services have certain services consolidated centrally (most commonly purchasing, contracting, or information technology). Outside those clearly defined areas, individual organizations retain autonomous operations and control. This model is depicted in Figure 3.3.

Affiliation with central services is an extension of the affiliation or regional delivery approaches, formalizing previously separate relationships into a central decision-making body. The long term viability of this model remains unproven; however, many organizations have selected this approach as a midpoint between a loose affiliation and the more structured corporate and regional delivery variants.

Information technology planning and management is a natural, logical function to locate at a central services organization, and affiliation with central services IDSs frequently choose to do that, either completely

Figure 3.3. Affiliation with Central Services IDS Model

Central Services Organization		Holding Company, Contractual or Joint- Venture Relationship

✓ Information technology
✓ Managed care services/TPA
✓ Management consulting
✓ Payer contracting
✓ Centralized business office
✓ Group purchasing

Hospital A	Payer	Physician Groups	Hospital B	Home Health/VNA

MANAGEMENT INTEGRATION: *MEDIUM TO HIGH*	PHYSICIAN INTEGRATION: *LOW TO MEDIUM*	IT INTEGRATION: *MEDIUM TO HIGH*
✓ Centralized in agreed areas; remainder is individual or facility controlled	✓ Loosely formalized or completely informal relationships	✓ Wide variation, from central data center offering uniform applications to centralized standards and purchase agreements

FINANCIAL INTEGRATION: *MEDIUM*	CONTINUUM-OF-CARE INTEGRATION: *MEDIUM TO HIGH*	
✓ CSO jointly funded, aligning risk and investment	✓ Target services through CSO or subcontracted or loose relationships	

standardizing IT planning, budgeting, and management functions or selecting critical core systems and technologies as "uniform" (such as networking, telecommunications, or Internet-related technologies) and decentralizing smaller decisions.

Corporate Ownership

The most tightly integrated of all current models, corporate IDSs have centralized management and decision making and may mandate organizational compliance with central policies and operations, as shown in Figure 3.4.

Figure 3.4. Corporate Ownership IDS Model

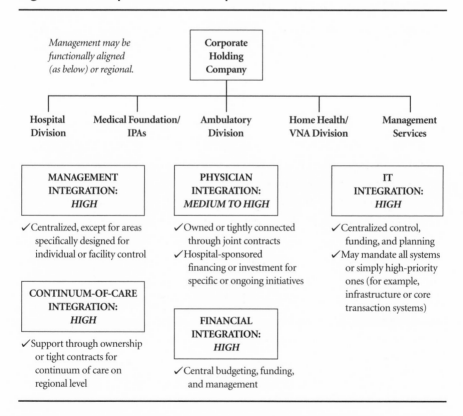

With tight central control, the corporate ownership model shares with regional delivery the advantage of stronger influence over IDS operations. Unlike regional delivery, however, breadth of geographical reach is clearly a key focus of the organization.

Corporate models can generally succeed at more complicated IT initiatives than other IDSs, primarily due to the tighter connections between organizations and facilities, centralized financing, and stronger management controls. Specific applications or technologies might include a corporate extranet with broad functionality for staff, physicians, patients, or even trading partners or the implementation of an enterprisewide electronic medical record or clinical data repository.

The "Virtual" IDS: Group Purchasing and Membership Organizations

To some health care providers, IDS business models are not possible or desirable approaches to business structure and care delivery. Nearly every group purchasing collective and many provider-oriented membership organizations today offer some of the advantages of an IDS. Leveraged negotiations with suppliers of a system, technology, or product by such a group—a "virtual" IDS—allows these organizations to provide their members with valuable products or services at a discount. Even for a well-evolved IDS, participation in this kind of virtual organization may complement or extend its existing strategy.

The virtual IDS operates by aligning multiple organizations' economic incentives and providing participating entities with opportunities for collaboration (rather than integration). It is not an integrated delivery system in the strict sense of the phrase, but it does offer organizations some similar benefits. True integrated delivery systems inherently share broader organizational and strategic incentives, with a collective "enterprise" focus rather than an individual-entity one.

IDS Models: Summary

Each of the common approaches to structuring an integrated delivery system offers trade-offs in terms of flexibility, control, and strategic orientation. Clearly, as integration within the IDS increases, so does the ability of the organization to plan and achieve more complex IT-related ventures. Table 3.3 summarizes the four IDS models.

IDS INFORMATION TECHNOLOGY MANAGEMENT

The inherently larger and more complex scope of integrated delivery system organizations correspondingly weights related IT needs and challenges. Traditional data and information requirements—billing, scheduling, medical records—are complicated by the addition of increased patient volume and varied sites and types of care delivery.

In addition, conceptual shifts associated with IDS business requirements (for example, accepting continuum-of-care requirements for a capitated patient population) present still different core information technology requirements. Some of these needs might include connecting distant organizations via local area network (LAN), wide area network (WAN), or Internet technology; tracking cross-organizational patient encounters; creating a community master member index; and supporting more complex case management tools.

Core management and planning structures, once implemented, can effectively position an IDS to manage the larger scope and intricacy of IT requirements. Even then, however, there are unique IT challenges—basic and advanced—that each organization must overcome to succeed.

Management and Planning Structures

The level of centralized IT management is a critical decision in IDS information technology planning and deployment. The decision must be made which applications and technologies are managed most effectively and efficiently from a centralized location and what degree of regional site or facility autonomy is practical and cost-efficient.

Regardless of the degree of centralization, there are five core strategies that effectively foster and evolve information technology development at the IDS level. Together they focus member organizations on common

Table 3.3. IDS Model Summary

	Affiliation Model	Regional Delivery Model	Affiliation with Central Services Model	Corporate Ownership Model
How created	Contract, joint venture	Growth, merger, acquisition	Contract, joint venture, merger	Ownership, merger, acquisition
Examples	Evergreen Community Health Care (Kirkland, Washington)	Children's Health System (San Diego, California)	Baycare Health System (Clearwater, Florida), Catholic Health Care West (San Francisco, California)	Sharp Healthcare (San Diego, California), Kaiser Group Health (Seattle, Washington)
Overall integration	Low to medium	Medium	Medium	High
IT strategies	• Decision making and control at the local level • Little attempt to standardize systems or operations • Common projects with mutual benefit	• Decision making and control may be very centralized, may remain at entity level • Enterprise oversight of specific areas	• Decision making and control largely centralized • Enterprise oversight of specific areas; some standard systems may be adopted	• Centralized decision making and control • Enterprise oversight of all areas not specifically excepted to the regional or local level

Table 3.3. Continued

	Affiliation Model	Regional Delivery Model	Affiliation with Central Services Model	Corporate Ownership Model
Systems implications	• Data sharing (eligibility lookup, contracting) between entities	• Centralized data repository • Enterprise DSS • Intranet-extranet system	• Risk and contracting • Intranet-extranet system • Telecom, networking	• Common core systems • Longitudinal data sharing • Case management, disease management
Market acceptance	*Proven* as a transitional model; *unproven* as an end-stage organizational structure	*Proven*	*Unproven*; there have been multiple and broadly publicized failures of organizations adopting this approach	*Proven*

goals and objectives while allowing sufficient flexibility to preserve individual organizational interests and perspectives. The strategies are as follows:

- Create and use central and specialized IT governance bodies.
- Sponsor initiatives appropriate for the development stage of the IDS.
- Develop and use coordinated interim and long-range IT plans.
- Where it makes economic or service delivery sense, consider system and operations consolidations.
- Develop a core competency in IT financial and benefits realization management.

Create and Use Central and Specialized IT Governance Bodies. Through an enterprisewide IT steering committee (also known as an information systems steering committee, or ISSC), the chief information officer can define criteria for central, regional, and local IT decision making, as well as establish and validate an enterprise vision of technology direction, strategy, applications planning, budgeting, and project approval. When multiple organizations or entities within the IDS are involved in a project, the committee should also oversee implementation efforts and sequencing. It is very important that this governance body include representation from all IDS business and service units and that the composition include senior or executive-level decision makers.

With the advent of newer, less developed technologies (wireless applications, Internet, clinical systems, and so on), many IDSs are extending the use of governance bodies beyond a central ISSC. Increasingly common are specialized committees—groups convened for a limited time duration with a specific charge, such as the development of an e-health strategy or the study or implementation of an enterprisewide electronic medical record. These groups can also be used to deal with regional issues or to ensure sufficient involvement of key user constituencies (such as physicians).

Sponsor Initiatives Appropriate for the Development Stage of the IDS. Any IDS structural model can benefit from an early and continuing focus on projects and initiatives providing common or overwhelming benefit across the enterprise. Adopting this IDS (rather than the individual-entity) perspective can maximize operational efforts, efficiencies, and financial investments. Project teams should involve cross-entity membership to foster enterprisewide views and team development. These "wins"—early and often—can build a foundation culture and philosophy of success from which larger, more complex IT projects can be built.

The following are some common IDS systems, projects, and initiatives.

- *Early IDS:* WAN or LAN, common financial systems, common electronic mail

- *Midstage IDS:* Integration technologies, departmental system consolidations, enterprise-master patient index, clinical data repository, common case management and service line systems

- *Advanced IDS:* Uniform systems or tight data or system integration capabilities

Develop and Use Coordinated Interim and Long-Range IT Plans. Rapid change has become more the norm than the exception in information technology planning. It is particularly important for organizations in transition to consider the strategic issues relating to IT, develop and document a formal vision, and then form and *periodically and consistently update* operational goals for the IT function.

In today's market, with constant business distractions and competition for capital, it is remarkably easy to find organizations focusing almost exclusively on short-term, crisis-related issues. Long-range plans provide a consistent direction for aligning business with information technology, guiding application usage, achieving benefits and return on investment, and competently staffing and governing the IT function.

Where It Makes Economic or Service Delivery Sense, Consider System and Operations Consolidations. Cost and quality efficiencies can often be gained from standardizing systems, operational units, or technologies at the IDS level. In some instances (for example, system and hardware maintenance contracting), the failure to coordinate or consolidate IDS operations verges on financial irresponsibility.

Executing this strategy, however, often requires centralized decision-making control or extraordinary organizational buy-in. Some areas to examine for standardization include the following:

- Application systems (scheduling, registration, financials)

- Operational areas (data processing, data center, central business office, regional lab)

- Foundation or advanced technologies (Internet-intranet-extranet; use of electronic data interchange (EDI) to facilitate claims, payments, or general commerce)

Develop a Core Competency in IT Financial and Benefits Realization Management. With the increased IT budgets of the past decade have come greater organizational visibility and scrutiny. Capital-competitive, cost-conscious organizations *must* be able to see clear financial value from information technology investments.

One of the most clearly documented benefits of integrating is the ability to use economies of scale for financial benefit. Other key financial considerations IDS management should consider relating to IT include these:

- *Consolidating IDS capital and operating budgets.* True organizational spending and potential efficiencies gained on IT are difficult to measure if individual facilities or entities all maintain distinct budgets. Gaining the maximum benefits from group purchasing and economy-of-scale opportunities requires consolidated examination of spending and return.

- *Establishing an IT value program.* By projecting strategic benefits and labor and cost efficiencies and by documenting postimplementation results, IDS organizations can set clear and quantifiable expectations for IT value, as well as establish a prioritization schema for considering new initiatives. By setting a continuous focus on the *value* that information technology brings to the IDS, justifying budget expenditures becomes much easier.

- *Considering alternative IT management approaches.* "Nontraditional" arrangements such as leasing and outsourcing are currently enjoying a renaissance. Supported by advances in Internet and EDI technologies, application service providers (ASPs) and focused interim management "SWAT teams" may meet IDS needs both quickly and effectively. These approaches may prove particularly effective for organizations that need to meet new requirements rapidly or that have limited available capital.

No matter what the IDS model or how effective the management team, organizations will face certain challenges relating to information technology.

Common and Advanced Challenges

The challenges organizations face vary somewhat according to their IDS approach, management structure, and level of comfort with information technology. In the early stages of IDS formation, typical issues and challenges relate strongly to infrastructure, communications, management, and operations. Later, as the IDS comes together and consolidates operations, deeper issues relating to physician integration, large-scale data management, data analysis, and population health begin moving to the forefront.

Disparate Development Levels of IT Infrastructure. Affiliation, merger, and acquisition are the cornerstone of IDS formation. In forming an IDS, providers must make a number of key decisions, including what components of care to incorporate into the IDS and what structure the new organization should assume.

From an IT perspective, rarely do organizations come together with the same systems, technologies, and operations. Far more commonly, completely disparate infrastructures exist and must be reconciled at least in part.

There are three common approaches:

1. *Completely standardize.* Application systems are replaced, with selection choices mandated or tightly restricted to a small number of "preferred vendors." This approach offers significant IT management benefits and eases long-term data capture and analysis; however, *significant* organizational and cultural resistance can make it difficult to implement.

2. *Standardize clusters.* This approach is becoming increasingly common as organizations recognize the cost benefits inherent in a manageable number of applications and technologies. Using this strategy, organizations standardize on a single vendor across a particular type of system. By grouping, say, patient administrative systems—billing, accounts receivable, scheduling, ADT (admission, discharge, and transfer), utilization review, quality assurance, and administrative medical records—at a single vendor, organizations can achieve many of the benefits of standard systems, reduce data interface requirements, and still achieve greater flexibility than if they pursued complete standardization.

3. *Maintain separate operations.* This approach, while failing to capture the obvious benefits of integration, provides for the maintenance of separate control and decision making by organizations within the IDS. For affiliation model IDSs, separate operations may in fact be maintained for quite some time before any wide consolidation is even attempted.

The Expanded Organization. At the IDS level, the information technology department must expand its definition of the end user, considering a much broader range of end users in their planning and support activities.

In some IDS structures, IT staff are asked to plan and support infrastructure for organizations that may not actually be owned or controlled by the IDS (for example, physician practices, home health services, or retail pharmacies).

Clearly, as today's business and IT managers are asked to support dissimilar business lines, organizations, and users in multiple locations, staffing models must reflect this increased diversity. The following are increasingly important pieces in the "IT skill set":

- Telecommunications and networking experience

- Operational experience with information technology in markets other than hospitals

- Experience in advanced technologies (including Internet-intranet-extranet systems, e-commerce, and e-health), data security, and working with very large databases or data sets

- Clinical and business process redesign skills, including change management capabilities

Cultural Implications of Merger. Consistently, organizations underestimate the time, energy, and difficulty of bringing together organizations with established infrastructures, operations, and cultural environments. It is dangerous to assume that just because separate entity management structures commit to a shared vision, individuals, groups, and departments within each entity will automatically fall in line. More than one IDS formed through merger has failed as a direct result of this "culture clash."

Although some issues cannot be avoided, several steps can be taken to manage the issues arising from merging unique organizations:

- *Appropriate planning and analysis before the merger or acquisition.* Organizations planning a merger or acquisition must clearly analyze the respective organizations; probable problems and issues should be identified and planned for—if not before the merger, then *as early as possible* in the IDS formation process. Such planning should consider the overall goals and objectives of the organizational merger and articulate possible approaches (including advantages and disadvantages) to IT planning, management, and operations for the new organization.

- *Clear management planning.* If layoffs are inevitable or if centralization is going to occur, the more prepared management is to deal with the inevitable difficulties, the more smoothly the transition will go.

- *Commitment to the new vision.* Management promotion, staff education, and setting clear goals and expectations will all contribute to the development of a new (and, ideally, improved) organizational culture.

SUMMARY

Despite significant discussion and much trial and error, there remain many flavors of integrated delivery systems, each adopting individual, local levels of consolidation and integrated activities. There have been successes and failures with each model, and the "right" way to be an IDS has not yet, and may never, become clear.

Planning and maintaining IT in support of existing and emerging IDS models requires that executives address a broad base of IT user management, control, and planning requirements consistently and comprehensively. The vision, purpose, strategic direction, and near-term requirements of the IDS clearly should drive major IT investment decisions. Failure to identify and align IDS vision with IT properly can result in a lack of essential IT capabilities and a failure to provide necessary support for business and medical service activities.

CHAPTER 4

The Systems Life Cycle

No technology has an indefinite life span. Over time, both hardware and software become outdated, increasingly unreliable, and expensive to maintain—this is true of the most advanced and complex supercomputer as well as the simplest electronic coffeemaker. Effectively maintaining health care information technology investments requires organizations to monitor and manage systems and hardware, periodically making the decision to reinvest or replace.

As health care has developed and adopted new and emerging technologies, it has become abundantly clear that not all technologies follow a single life cycle. Planning horizons, development cycles, and external influences all shape the life and utility of a technology. Identifying and managing this systems life cycle in a consistent, logical, and disciplined way can ensure and extend the effective life span of many IT investments.

THE SYSTEMS LIFE CYCLE

Traditionally, discussions of the systems development life cycle have followed a linear path through four discrete stages—strategic planning, vendor selection and system development, systems implementation, and maintenance. Every four to five years, the cycle would restart as the organization reexamined its current state and desired future direction.

This traditional approach, however, does not fully capture the complex interactions between business and technology and lags behind today's accelerated business-to-technology alignment and benefit cycles.

An astonishing breadth and depth of technological choice is available to today's health care organization. Many of these technologies have similar life cycles, allowing for the creation of IT management "tracks"— groups of applications and technologies that can be planned for and administered collectively. There are four such tracks, and effective planning considers organizational requirements in each area.

- *Infrastructure.* Networking and foundation technologies, these systems provide the basic building blocks of intra- and interorganizational communications.

- *Core transaction systems.* These are the basic systems used in daily operations, including administrative, financial, and baseline clinical functions.

- *Strategic systems (including decision support).* These are the systems that incorporate expert rules, artificial intelligence, or some other type of intelligent analysis of raw data, assisting in better administrative, financial, or clinical decision making.

- *Emerging technologies.* This category encompasses new, unproven technologies that fundamentally change operations or workflow, including such advanced technologies as workflow, fully functional electronic medical records, and telemedical and telehealth applications.

Life Cycle Approach

The Business to Technology Alignment approach is one way to view the systems life cycle. It focuses on identifying and exploiting the interdependencies between business practices and technology potential, allowing health care organizations to take maximum advantage of their unique organizational, market, and technological characteristics. Figure 4.1 provides an illustration of this approach.

Figure 4.1. Business to Technology Alignment Methodology

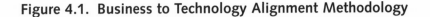

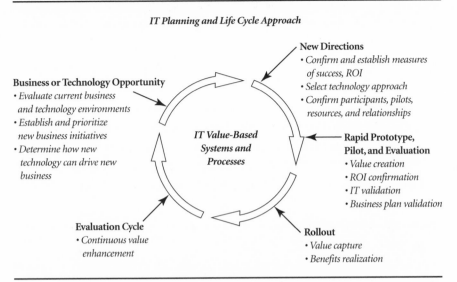

IT Planning and Life Cycle Approach

New Directions
- *Confirm and establish measures of success, ROI*
- *Select technology approach*
- *Confirm participants, pilots, resources, and relationships*

Business or Technology Opportunity
- *Evaluate current business and technology environments*
- *Establish and prioritize new business initiatives*
- *Determine how new technology can drive new business*

IT Value-Based Systems and Processes

Rapid Prototype, Pilot, and Evaluation
- *Value creation*
- *ROI confirmation*
- *IT validation*
- *Business plan validation*

Evaluation Cycle
- *Continuous value enhancement*

Rollout
- *Value capture*
- *Benefits realization*

Note: Copyright © 2000 Information Technology Optimizers, Inc. Business to Technology Alignment is a service mark of Health Care Investment Visions LLC.

The value of this approach lies in the way it facilitates best outcomes in three critical areas:

- It integrates business and technology opportunity planning.
- It emphasizes the search for "pivot" opportunities. Pivots are ways the organization can quickly capture and demonstrate value, market share, or product benefits and consequently position for change in fundamental architecture and IT approach.[1]
- It emphasizes the creation of organizational value through rapid implementation and ROI cycles wherever possible.

---

[1]For an excellent discussion of the importance and relevance of assimilating business opportunities and technology potential, see Bernard H. Boar, *The Art of Strategic Planning for Information Technology* (New York: Wiley, 1993).

Life Cycle Influences

The effective life span of every technology is affected by outside forces (technological change, user requirements, regulatory and management trends), although the extent and nature of the impact may vary. Changes in health care business requirements can create new markets (or eliminate old ones) for software applications. In the 1980s, the emergence of the prospective payment system and diagnosis-related groupings (DRGs) for provider reimbursement drove the adoption of a new generation of managed care reimbursement systems. Other changing business requirements might include increased consumer demand for health-related information or more sophisticated payroll and cafeteria benefits requirements.

A number of other factors, together with unique organizational needs and characteristics, determine the useful life span of any particular technology.

Evolving Outsourcing and Alternative Pricing Models. Vendors with adapted outsourcing structures and creative pricing models offer increasingly attractive benefits to provider organizations. Outsourcers and application service providers (an updated, current-day evolution of shared systems) are offering rapid response, compelling flexibility, and defined accountability for information systems and technology goals. These models reduce the capital requirements for obtaining system functionality, giving organizations the ability to reinvest immediately as new and more robust applications emerge.

Hardware Price and Performance. The price and performance of hardware continues to increase exponentially. Older hardware technologies are giving way to a miniaturization of electrical components, as well as a reduction in size, facilities requirements (such as air conditioning and power), and movable parts (such as disk drives). Also, new types of hardware (such as optical computers) are emerging as viable alternatives to more traditional equipment. As such, hardware vendors have an incentive to pressure user organizations to upgrade hardware continually. To user organizations, this ongoing trend means that hardware investments should be made only when required (for example, when two-year maintenance costs begin to exceed upgrade costs).

Viability of Internet-Enabled Applications. Internet-enabled systems (hosted by the health care organization or an application services provider) can run on any hardware device capable of sustaining an Internet connection, offering organizations the flexibility of a client-server architecture without the high cost of maintenance. As vendor organizations continue to develop and roll out Internet-enabled applications, health care organizations should consider fundamental shifts in their approach to systems architecture and IT management. As trading partners and affiliated health care organizations develop Internet-centric infrastructures, the pressure on health care organizations to develop and sustain their own capabilities in this area will continue to increase.

Software Vendor Incentives. Although a significant portion of software vendor revenue comes from maintenance contracts for existing software, traditional software vendors also depend on the license fees associated with the sale of new software modules or upgrades. Consequently, they have incentives to redevelop their systems periodically with new technology and design parameters. Assuming a reasonable level of responsibility and quality assurance on the part of the vendor, providers who reinvest in significantly enhanced systems can capture benefits from newer design and programming techniques as well as expanded functionality and benefits.

Changing Technology, Design, and Programming Techniques. Technology and technology development approaches, like health care business requirements, are continually changing. Today's software developers are taking advantage of newer, faster, and cheaper ways of building systems and technologies—ways that allow them to pass along price incentives or build more advanced capabilities into their systems. Perhaps counterintuitively, the increasing standardization of software applications often works to *lengthen* the life of current technology. Most software vendors are developing systems that can potentially interconnect with other existing systems, providing users with greater capabilities and flexibility of choice.

Increasing Dependencies Among Application Systems, Networks, and Telecommunications Technologies. As information technology grows increasingly sophisticated, incorporating advanced capabilities such as e-commerce and data exchange, considerable advantage flows to information systems that work well with existing network and telecommunications platforms. Health care has made significant progress in adhering to standardized network and telecommunications protocols, less so with standardized electronic data interchange transactions. The passage of the Health Insurance Portability and Accountability Act (HIPAA), mandating standardized transaction sets, will eventually stimulate progress in this area, allowing further advancement in application system, network, and telecommunications data exchange.

Life Cycle Risks

The varied risks and complexities of the technology "tracks" discussed earlier give rise to different strategies and considerations during planning, vendor selection, system implementation, and ongoing maintenance. Table 4.1 discusses these differences.

INFORMATION TECHNOLOGY PLANNING

Traditionally, health care organizations have conducted business planning and IT planning separately. But the two processes provide each other with critical input and driving forces and should be conducted concurrently whenever possible. Figure 4.2 gives an overview of such a combined process.

The CEO's Guide to Health Care Information Systems

IT planning initiatives provide the opportunity for health care organizations to assess their information technology status and performance against industry standards, best practices, and current or future expected business requirements. Based on the outcome of that assessment, the organization can formulate strategies and define a plan to ensure that future IT investments are targeted to meet key needs and objectives. Although it remains possible to define a five-year vision, the rapid pace of change in both health care and IT has shortened the length of effective tactical planning. Today, beyond a two- to three-year time frame, forecasting with any reasonable accuracy is difficult, if not impossible.

The Planning Process

Done well, strategic information technology planning is an ongoing, dynamic process. Ideally, an organization develops an initial long-range plan and executes periodic updates and changes. As plan objectives are reached, their actual impact should be compared to the expected effects, and new objectives should be set.

There are a number of critical factors the plan should consider:

- The composition and complexity of the organization, including management team capabilities and level of support, organizational tolerance for risk, and level of IT competency within the organization

- Organizational expectations for quantifiable return from information systems and information technology investments

- Established organizational business and medical services goals

- Established and "in process" organizational systems and technologies

- The surrounding health care marketplace

- Available technologies—both in and beyond health care—that might be adopted in new or unusual ways or that might drive a new way of doing business (for example, some organizations have adopted the use of pager technology to improve patient compliance with specific drug regimens)

Table 4.1. Life Cycle Considerations

Technology Type	Planning	Selection	Implementation	Maintenance
Infrastructure technology	• Largely driven by capacity needs and expected growth	• Commodity market, price sensitivity • Vendor reliability a key concern	• Down time must be minimized or eliminated • Third parties performing implementation may not be formally associated with equipment vendor	• Price and performance increase rapidly
Core systems (clinical, administrative, financial)	• Mostly mature market • Driven by replacement cycles	• Best of breed or cluster approach? • Handful of dominant vendors	• Basic vendor plans are tested and proven • Focus on task and milestone accountability	• Does reinvestment analysis show continued value to organization? • Is vendor appropriately upgrading system to meet new needs?

Table 4.1. Continued

Technology Type	Planning	Selection	Implementation	Maintenance
Strategic systems (decision support, clinical protocols)	• Driven by business, financial, and clinical organizational strategies	• Content knowledge of selection team important	• Can require significant process reengineering • Success requires more cooperation between vendor and provider organization	• Shorter cycles, rapidly changing marketplace
Emerging technologies (workflow, electronic medical records)	• Requires significant risk tolerance	• Health care organization assumes significant risk • Likely to involve heavy customization	• Reengineering of organizational processes is *essential* • Requires strong partnership between vendor and health care organization	• Formal benefits quantification is critical to judging success

Figure 4.2. Value-Based Systems and Processes

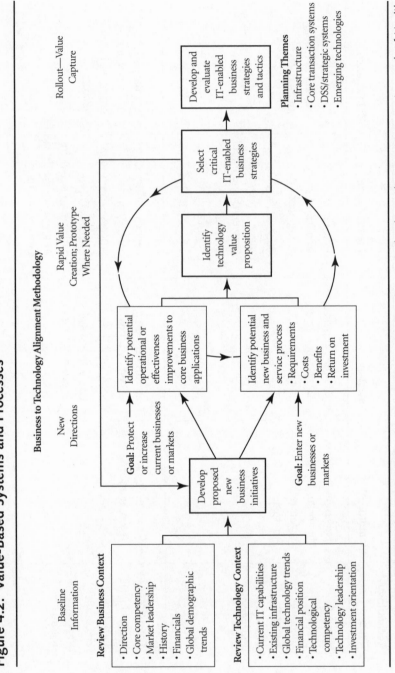

Business to Technology Alignment Methodology

Baseline Information | New Directions | Rapid Value Creation; Prototype Where Needed | Rollout—Value Capture

Review Business Context
- Direction
- Core competency
- Market leadership
- History
- Financials
- Global demographic trends

Review Technology Context
- Current IT capabilities
- Existing infrastructure
- Global technology trends
- Financial position
- Technological competency
- Technology leadership
- Investment orientation

Develop proposed new business initiatives

Goal: Protect or increase current businesses or markets

Goal: Enter new businesses or markets

Identify potential operational or effectiveness improvements to core business applications

Identify potential new business and service process
- Requirements
- Costs
- Benefits
- Return on investment

Identify technology value proposition

Select critical IT-enabled business strategies

Develop and evaluate IT-enabled business strategies and tactics

Planning Themes
- Infrastructure
- Core transaction systems
- DSS/strategic systems
- Emerging technologies

It is important to remember that during the course of a planning period, a health care organization's situation and needs might shift. The shift might be organizational (a major change in the strategic business or medical service vision of the facility), market-oriented (emergence of a new and vigorous competitor, a significant change in consumer or patient behaviors), regulatory (major shift in Medicare reimbursement), or technological (new technology application that solves the security problem of storing and sending clinical data over the Internet). Indeed, part of developing a plan should be to anticipate such changes and their possible effects on the institution.

Basic Planning Guidelines. There are a number of basic guidelines that can facilitate effective IT planning.

- Articulate how all technology supports the organization's mission.
- Build the systems vision on a strong, flexible technology foundation.
- Establish firm expectations and stick with them. Make systems decisions because defined benefits are expected. Keep requirements in focus at all times.
- Focus on information as an *organizational* resource (rather than a departmental or entity resource). Make user business and operational needs of prime importance, and incorporate user training and retraining as an essential component of IT management.
- Recognize and manage risk. It is inevitable.
- Remember that a plan is just a blueprint. To meet organizational needs, it must set a clear vision while also establishing achievable goals, milestones, and timelines. Yet it must also be flexible enough to change along the course of the plan.

Process Milestones. Formulating a strategic plan is not an exact science. Each plan must reflect the unique vision, structure, expectations, and capabilities of the sponsoring organization. Still, consistently conducting key tasks and activities ensures that required information is collected and analyzed and provides an adequate level of quality assurance for the end product. Exhibit 4.1 lists the critical process milestones for an IT planning initiative.

From Plan to Action

Through the long-range planning process, most organizations are able to come up with one or more pivot opportunities (areas or technologies in which considerable immediate value can accrue to the organization), as well as areas where new technologies can provide a base for a future, broader range of applications. In executing a long-range plan, there are a series of action steps that can identify the most effective solution to meet organizational needs:

1. *Organizational analysis and feasibility evaluation.* How will current systems, processes, and work structures be affected by the new system or technology? Will the current infrastructure support its use? What specific requirements, features, and functions will the new system or technology be required to support?

2. *Market availability and development approach.* Do fully developed, "off the shelf" solutions exist in the area under consideration? Will the organization support the added risk of custom development, or will a packaged system be purchased from one or more vendors?

3. *External data collection and analysis.* Information is solicited from potential vendors and development partners, and their supplied data are analyzed against organizational requirements and preferences.

4. *Solution selection.* The organization chooses one or more vendors or partners.

5. *Contract negotiation.* Pricing and task responsibilities are formalized, including a detailed implementation plan to map task requirements, execution, responsibilities, and system formation. Also at this time, any additional network or telecommunication enhancement needs are identified.

Exhibit 4.1. IT Planning Process Milestones

- Develop project plan, resource schedule, and team roster.
- Initiate executive and user functions. Form advisory and oversight committees, develop charters and mission statements, and begin educational efforts.
- Gather baseline technology information: voice, data, and networks, including architecture, pending and planned projects, budgets, and staffing.
- Gather baseline business information: business and medical service plans, organizational goals and objectives, auditor reports, regional market area competitor information.
- Review business context. Align known and potential business and medical service strategies with IT requirements, develop proposed ROI expectations and guidelines, and conduct exploration and brainstorming with executive and user committees.
- Review technology context. Formulate IT strategy to address core system deficiencies and to improve core business functions, review expandability versus expendability of current systems, and conduct exploration and brainstorming with executive and user committees.
- Develop IT strategies, tactics, and value proposition. Identify alternative technology approaches and technologies within value context; project estimated costs, benefits, and risks associated with each alternative; and document findings.
- Select alternative strategies. Balance the developed alternatives against organizational priorities; evaluate expandability versus expendability of each and the roles of Internet-intranet-extranet, e-health, and organizational service lines.
- Develop an IT management plan. Expand and conduct operational planning for selected alternatives and strategies. The plan should, at a minimum, contain the following sections:
  Executive summary
  Vision, architecture, and direction overview
  Benefit attainment guidelines and plan
  Multiyear capital and operations budgets
  Information technology function and department plan
- Review and approve plan.

6. *System implementation.* Newly purchased systems or technologies are licensed, detail implementation plans are formed, and the process of changing systems (or implementing a new system) is closely managed by the organization.

7. *Postimplementation review and reinvestment analysis.* At this point, the actual return of an investment is measured against projected benefits. For existing systems, the continued value (versus the value potentially offered by a new investment) is validated.

The first two steps are extensions of the long-range planning process, focusing the organization more clearly on the possibilities and "fit" between a system or technology and the organization. Steps 3 through 5 (data collection, solution selection, and contract negotiation) are part of selecting an IT software or services provider. The selected system is actualized in step 6 (system implementation), and step 7 (review and reinvestment analysis) closes the loop by comparing projected to actual benefits and positioning the organization for future goals and objectives.

Feasibility Evaluation and Market Availability

Prior to implementing a technology within a health care organization (particularly one new to the organization, a strategic system, or an unproven, emerging technology), executive leadership must feel comfortable that the technology will succeed. In some circumstances, this is a relatively simple matter; for example, the benefits and success potential of an electronic admission, discharge, and transfer system are straightforward and easily articulated.

Other technologies are not so clear. A consumer-oriented, Web-based personal health record is new, expensive, and (so far) unproven. Examining the feasibility of a technology before committing to an IT investment accomplishes two key goals:

• It validates the potential value of the technology to the organization.

• It creates a realistic technology development plan to manage risk and maximize success.

The extensiveness of a feasibility study varies considerably by type of technology, of course, but such a study should include at least all of the following information:

- Market conditions (local, regional, and national)
- Executive readiness to accept and support new technology
- Organizational structure and services
- Application opportunities for the new technology—how it can and will be used throughout the health care enterprise
- Technology development and deployment status
- Potential impact of the new technology—how existing workflows and processes will be affected through implementation
- Cost-benefit and return-on-investment analysis
- Relevant vendors
- Recommended strategies for implementation

Upon completion of the study, the organization can proceed to selecting a software or service provider that offers the new technology or has the capabilities to develop or co-develop it.

SELECTING AN IT SOFTWARE OR SERVICE PROVIDER

Once the information technology plan has been completed and accepted and a development approach has been selected, organizations move into the next phase of operationalizing their IT vision by selecting a vendor or partner. The capital and operational dollars at stake in these decisions are rarely small—health care IT purchases can run into the millions of dollars, and a failed selection can cost an organization time, energy, and momentum in addition to money.

An effective selection process, whether for a packaged software product, a development partner, or a service provider, incorporates enough structure to collect, evaluate, and measure the potential offering against organizational needs.

Data Collection and Analysis

There are a number of schools of thought about asking for information from potential vendors or development partners.

The *request for proposal* (RFP) offers vendors an extremely comprehensive listing of potential system features and functions, asking for a binary yes or no response to each item. It also requires vendors to submit a detailed and binding price quotation for the sought applications and services. Up to three hundred pages long, responses to this document provide health care organizations with a total look at the robustness of systems under consideration. The RFP is the highest-cost way to collect vendor information, for both the health care organization and the technology product or service supplier.

Another potential information gathering tool, the *request for information* (RFI), is considerably shorter, generally focusing on a particular vendor's background, the basic product description, and a series of qualitative questions about product and service capabilities. Vendors are typically asked to provide pricing guidelines (how they would calculate the purchase price) rather than a binding price quote. This is the lowest-cost approach; it also provides the least amount of data.

A third type of data collection approach offers a compromise between the RFP and the RFI. Increasing numbers of organizations are using a *vendor system proposal* (VSP) to initiate selection projects. The VSP mixes the approaches of the other two tools, providing binary detail on organizationally identified "critical" areas while leaving other areas to use the qualitative or essay approach. Vendors are asked to provide cost-benefit justification for their system, through best practice or benchmark reporting, in addition to as specific a financial quote as possible with the information they have.

In determining the approach to adopt, health care organizations should consider what type of system they are planning to select, its critical importance to the overall organization, the type of technology (for example, emerging technologies are often not yet well developed, meaning that presenting detailed binary questions about features and functions may yield untrustworthy answers), and the overall vendor selection approach. Exhibit 4.2 details some distinctions between the three tools.

Whichever approach an organization decides to use, the data collection tool should accomplish a number of things.

First, it should provide recipients with sufficient detail as to the health care organization's current structure, information technology vision, and future plans to evaluate how the vendor's offering can best meet the health care organization's specific requirements. Failing to provide potential vendors with adequate detail in this area is analogous to asking for directions to the airport while refusing to reveal your current location. One of the most frequently heard complaints from technology suppliers is the incredible lack of detail health care organizations are willing to share while expecting tremendous detail in return, perfectly aligned to the organization's needs.

Exhibit 4.2. Choosing a Data Collection Tool

When to Use a Request for Proposal

- When the technology being selected is established and fully developed
- When there is little variability between offering vendors
- When the organization has enough time to fully evaluate potential technologies
- When the organization needs strong contract protection from the selected vendor (by incorporating RFP response as a contract attachment)

When to Use a Request for Information

- When the organization requires information to support a feasibility analysis
- When the end users of the system being selected are a small and clearly defined group

When to Use a Vendor System Proposal

- When requesting any kind of developmental relationship with vendor (alpha, beta, joint venture)
- When investigating emerging technologies

Second, it should yield from recipients enough specific detail that the organization can understand the vendor, its company vision, its future plans, its core technology, the system, and the pricing proposed.

Third, it should yield from recipients enough specific detail that "vaporware" (undeveloped, unproven software) becomes immediately recognizable.

Finally, it should not indulge in unnecessary detail for the sake of detail. Recognize that extensive RFPs require significant effort, analysis, and review by both vendor and health care organization staff, for sometimes incremental return. If the health care organization's critical focus is on vendors' timelines for making Web-based front ends generally available to users, *that* is the question that belongs in the document, not "Discuss the five-year detail of your research and development plans."

Exhibit 4.3 provides a sample table of contents for a vendor system proposal.

Note that many vendors have staff dedicated to answering inquiries from potential clients and often use "boilerplate" information to answer common questions. To some extent, such responses may prove adequate for health care organization requirements. In other circumstances, the text will be too vague or slightly off-target. The more clearly the provider can state its information needs, the more specifically the vendor should be able to answer.

Vendor Demonstrations

System demonstrations can prove remarkably effective or exceedingly tedious. Given free reign, a vendor's demonstration staff (who almost always know the systems they demonstrate in remarkable detail) can spend hours showing bells and whistles while completely avoiding major design or performance flaws.

For that reason, it is crucially important that health care organizations clearly structure demonstration times, giving each vendor an opportunity to show off its system but maintaining adequate quality checks to uncover critical system or performance defects. A "scripted"

Exhibit 4.3. Typical Contents of a Vendor System Proposal

- *Proposal Deadline and Contacts.* When and where responses are to be directed; what individual is responsible for answering questions specific to the VSP.

- *Confidentiality and Contracting.* A statement acknowledging the confidential and proprietary nature of both the VSP and the responses provided by vendors. This section also typically includes a notice to respondents that issuance of the VSP does not obligate the health care organization to contract with anyone. Finally, if the HCO intends to incorporate the response into a final contract, that information will also be provided.

- *Completion Instructions.* Special formats, sections, and other requirements that vendors must comply with to be considered.

- *Organizational and Project Background.* Sufficient background detail about the HCO that vendors can effectively tailor their responses. Organizational size, patient volumes, and current systems overviews are provided here. Also in this section is a description of the project under consideration—key objectives, goals, and future visions.

- *Vendor Qualifications.* This section inquires as to the vendor organization's general background and experience, financial status, current clients, standard service, contract, and implementation plans.

- *Proposed Solutions.* In one or more sections, vendors are asked to detail their proposed solutions; binary as well as qualitative detail is requested.

- *Best Practices and Return on Investment.* Case studies, management engineering analyses, and other evidence of benefits that the proposed system may offer the health care organization.

- *Pricing and Support.* Specific questions regarding costing and technical support. Cost sections are usually standardized across vendors (to ease comparison across respondents).

demonstration, directing vendors to walk through specified system features, can also keep participants focused on important system qualities rather than being sidetracked by a charismatic demonstrator or a particularly nifty feature. Another benefit to scripting demonstrations is that it provides a benchmark of ease of system use—a comfortable user of the current system can be timed running through the script, tracking keystrokes, number of screens, and ease of use compared to those of the systems under consideration.

When There Is No Product to Buy: Information Technology Services

Selecting a service vendor is, by nature, a more qualitative process than choosing a tangible product. Whether the organization is selecting a product development partner, a consulting firm, or a systems integrator, these selections, of necessity, require a more qualitative judgment by provider executives. The following are some key considerations when selecting service providers.

Supervising Executive. Who is the individual in charge of the engagement? Is he or she of a caliber of experience that inspires confidence in the vendor's ability to complete the job? Does this person respond to organizational requests for clarification, assistance, or other contacts? Is the sales executive actually part of the work project, or will new individuals be charged with maintaining the relationship? Does the individual leading the vendor project team fit into the provider organizational culture? Is the project leader a "visionary"—able to focus, direct, and execute plans—or more operational? (Which is preferable depends on the project as well as the leadership capabilities of the provider organization.)

Relevant References. Can the organization provide references (including clients of a similar size and composition) where the proposed project or a similar one was completed successfully? Will this project be handled by the same staff?

Skill Mix of the Proposed Team. Vendor organization experience is important, but the qualifications of the actual project team matter as well.

What skills do the proposed team members have? Have key individuals been interviewed? What guarantees is the vendor willing to provide that the team being proposed will actually be the team that completes the project?

Cost, Cost Protections, and Mutual Incentives. How clearly can the vendor articulate the project components? Are mutual expectations, milestones, and success metrics clearly defined? Is the vendor willing to build price protections and "at risk" performance clauses into the contract (for example, stating that project cost is a flat fee or a "not to exceed" figure or that the payment schedule for accepted service milestones is incentive-based)? Are expected service performance levels clearly defined? Are the terms for bonus or incentive payments clearly spelled out?

After Selection: Negotiating a Favorable Contract

An effective vendor contracting process breaks down into three phases: prenegotiation research and screening, negotiations, and postcontracting measurement. Exhibit 4.4 identifies the key tasks in each phase.

Exhibit 4.4. Phases of Information Technology Contracting

Prenegotiation Research and Screening

- Identify "deal breakers"—critical contracting terms.

- Identify areas of high risk for the provider organization, and develop contracting strategies to minimize them.

- Set expectations with vendors.

- Investigate other providers' experience with vendors.

- Draw up a contract issues document.

Negotiations

- Identify likely points of contention, and address them early in negotiations.

- Use the contract issues document to track progress and resolution.

Postcontracting Measurement

- Monitor contracted obligations.

- Verify milestone completion.

- Conduct random contract audits.

- Track and report vendor service obligations.

Information technology contracts can be complex, often with literally hundreds of items addressed. Here are some general guidelines for coming to terms with a vendor.

- Never sign a vendor's standard agreement.

- Come to terms with financial arrangements as early in the negotiations as possible. Discussion about additional software, software options, extended warranties, and other matters will continue throughout the negotiation process; however, major pricing issues should emerge early in discussions and be resolved. Particularly for emerging technologies, vendors are often flexible on pricing structures and willing to consider nontraditional or at-risk arrangements, including product revenue sharing and equity positions.

- Insist that the vendor negotiator has sufficient authority to come to an agreement. A constant refrain of "Let me get back to you on that" is a sure sign that the wrong representative is at the table. Similarly, be certain that the individuals representing the health care organization have the authority to make commitments for the group. However, it can be beneficial to preserve the very top decision maker (ordinarily the CEO) for critical, extraordinary, or other "deal-breaking" agreements, providing the health care organization some amount of breathing space should negotiations become stalled or intense around a particular issue.

- Be certain the vendor knows you are willing to walk away from the table if you are unable to come to agreement within a reasonable period of time.

- Keep the negotiating team small (three or less); never allow disagreement at the table among team members. If differences of opinion arise, resolve them privately.

- Remember that the end goal is not just to buy hardware and software. Rather, it is to buy a successful, well-installed system that effectively meets the needs of the organization.

- Communicate expectations to potential vendors clearly and, if possible, in advance.

Many health care organizations now issue acquisition guidelines before negotiations start, alerting vendors to key organization desires and issues in advance. The guidelines often cover such points as these:

- License, warranty, and system maintenance
- Permitted users
- Acceptance testing and payment schedules
- VSP, RFP, or RFI inclusion (Making the vendor's original proposal and representations made during the selection process part of the final contract may prove effective in reining in brash vendor promises during the evaluation process. Note, however, that most vendors now insist on the right to review and change all representations made, including the VSP response, prior to inclusion.)
- Implementation planning
- Travel and out-of-pocket expense limits
- Network requirements and standards
- Response time guarantees for end users as well as for overall system performance
- Hardware requirements
- Price and payment terms, including any algorithms, formulas, or service thresholds being used to calculate price
- Technology protection (If a vendor discontinues a product line or migrates to an incompatible hardware platform, the contract should provide for price or source code guarantees to ensure continued operations.)
- Legal options for project and contract termination (Including this in the contract can protect the organization in the case of an unforeseen organizational event, such as a merger or acquisition.)
- Intellectual property and ownership rights (This is an issue that health care organizations must deal with contractually, particularly in two areas. First, as health care organizations more frequently co-develop applications with software developers, the long-term rights and

responsibilities of each organization toward the developed product must be articulated. Second, as providers send increasingly larger amounts of patient and organizational-specific data across privately owned vendor networks, a number of software developers are claiming rights or derivative rights to use those data in other ways.)

It is usually in a health care organization's best interests to negotiate with more than one vendor during system selection. Assuming more than one vendor meets organizational quality standards, this approach preserves options until a contract offering the greatest value to the organization can be obtained.

An organized approach to contract negotiations is absolutely crucial to ensuring that important issues are not overlooked. Studying the vendor's standard contract in advance and preparing a contract issues document (CID) can help keep discussions focused on the issues most important to the health care organization. As issues are dealt with, the provider team can note their resolution directly on the CID. Part of a sample CID is shown in Table 4.2.

SYSTEM IMPLEMENTATION

System implementation is by far the most detail-oriented component of the systems life cycle. Installing a health care application system can be a large and complex undertaking, requiring six months to a year or more of concerted effort by organizational staff, consultants, and vendor implementation teams. New, different, or unproven technologies can require even greater effort by the health care organization to plan and implement, as they frequently require more significant process and workflow changes.

A structured implementation effort has the following characteristics:

• It outlines essential tasks, schedules, responsibilities, and budgets.

• It incorporates a detailed examination of data, network, information, and telecommunications needs associated with the new technology.

Table 4.2. Sample Contract Issues Document

Issue	Desired Outcome	Importance	Resolution
Software maintenance payments begin at time of contract signature	Software maintenance should begin upon final system acceptance	Medium	
Contract specifies payment in full prior to final system acceptance	Payment should be milestone-based, with a final payment (a "holdback") for system acceptance	High	
Vendor claims ownership of data that flows over vendor network	Distribution of data without health care organization approval is prohibited; contract should clearly name HCO as data "owner"	Deal breaker	
Vendor does not offer a toll-free help line for end users	Physicians should have low-cost or cost-free access to technical support	Low to medium	
Contract has no financial incentives for vendor	Part of the total cost should be tied to successful rollout or implementation—after x users are on the system, vendor receives y amount of payment	High/deal breaker	

- It redesigns processes to maximize the benefits of the technology and the quantitative return on investment achieved by the organization.
- A single individual is charged with coordinating the efforts of all participants involved in the planning and implementation process (senior management, IS staff, end users and managers, the system vendor, and any others).
- It involves end users and IS staff closely in the site-specific system design. While the majority of vendors will offer a plan to implement their systems, those plans do not take into account the unique organizational requirements for changing or creating new processes.
- It incorporates quality management and early-warning and correction mechanisms, ensuring that issues and problems are documented clearly and immediately and are brought to the table for resolution with organizational senior management or the system vendor.

The inherent change involved in implementing a new system offers health care organizations the opportunity to significantly reengineer old or stale work processes. This opportunity also presents a formidable challenge. More than one system has failed because a health care organization did not take the time to develop adequate organizational buy-in to the new application. Here are some additional important success characteristics:

- Strong and determined organizational sponsorship
- Mutual incentives and aligned expectations between the system vendor and the health care organization, *incorporated into the purchase contract* (This typically includes a detailed implementation commitment— milestones, deliverables, contract holdbacks, schedules—delineating the clear responsibilities of both the vendor and the health care organization. Benefit goals and accountability measures for both sides are clearly documented.)
- Comprehensive implementation plans
- Adequate system acceptance testing
- Strong and well-planned end user training

• Appropriate time allowed for data conversion

• Minimal business and service disruptions

Most of these characteristics can be addressed in the implementation plan. Vendors frequently have a generic work plan they use when installing an application or technology. Though this is a very good starting point, health care organizations should always customize the plan to reflect their own unique circumstances. Exhibit 4.5 identifies some of the information that should be included in the implementation plan.

Exhibit 4.5. Components of a System Implementation Plan

• *Conversion Planning.* What information stored in the old system will be transferred into the new one? What information will be re-created for the new system?

• *Data Gathering.* New systems require files to be built, with patient types, physicians, payer listings, organizational contracts, and so on. What data will be necessary, where will they come from, and who will perform these tasks?

• *New Process Final Design and Future State.* What will workflow at the organization look like upon completion of the system installation?

• *System Building.* What resources will be assigned and accountable for completing required tasks (building the system tables, implementing the application, and so on)?

• *Training Requirements.* What level and approach of training will be required for end users and IS staff? How will it be completed in time to "go live"?

• *Cycle Testing Plans.* How will staff test the software prior to acceptance? It is crucial that each function of the software be tested after building files to be certain that the system is working correctly and that data were converted accurately.

• *Technical Specifications and Plans.* These include site, network, cabling, and communications plans to ensure that each site has the required hardware and equipment to run the system and perform its everyday operations. An equipment list should indicate which sites have what equipment.

After implementation, there is a period of organizational transition—end users adapt to new processes and gain comfort with the system (or don't), and previously unforeseen technical glitches may appear and be worked out. After a reasonable transition period, return on investment can be measured. As discussed in Chapter Two, organizations are taking a variety of approaches to ROI measurement, from detailed quantitative studies to qualitative or "best practices" analysis.

Conducting an ROI analysis for each new system or technology provides an important validation point for the organization, substantiating projected benefits, identifying unanticipated benefits, and generally setting baseline expectations for future returns. Far too many organizations fail to complete this critical activity. Another neglected step is a periodic reinvestment analysis, or an examination of when the benefits of an existing system begin to be outweighed by either the dollar costs required to maintain it or the opportunity costs of implementing a newer or more effective system.

SUMMARY

Effective information systems and technology planning is a frequently nonlinear, iterative process that requires significant management attention. The successful organization remains flexible in approach yet consistent in structure. Striking this balance allows room for innovation while ensuring consideration of core business system continuity, critical decision support information and requirements to meet quality standards, and return-on-investment expectations.

CHAPTER 5

Managing Health Care Information Technology

There is no "right" structure for an information technology function; a rich variety of management philosophies, organizational forms, and operational approaches are in use today. Delivery systems make a variety of decisions about degree of centralization, type of executive management, and functional organization that match the organization's charter, goals, and culture.

In general, however, an effective IT management program requires three distinct components: effective executive leadership, oversight and governance, and staff or departmental structure. Each component holds certain responsibilities and faces typical challenges; together, they interconnect to build the framework that supports effective information technology planning, implementation, and ongoing management.

There is no universal terminology for the information technology function. Historically called the data processing or the management information system (MIS) department, organizations today have adopted any number of other labels: information resources, information systems, information services, information management, information technology services. For simplicity of discussion, we will refer to the information services (IS) department.

EXECUTIVE LEADERSHIP

Over the past decade, as IT has assumed a more visible and more strategic role in many organizations, the role of the top IT executive has gained correspondingly greater importance. Today, while many organizations have committed to the position of chief information officer (CIO) as a senior management team participant, other organizations retain a line management structure and emphasis. These organizations may term the position an IS director or may use the CIO title with a reporting structure (often to the chief financial officer) that does not give the position equal status with other senior executives.

This inconsistent industry view of the CIO arises somewhat from the inconsistent view of health care IT—is it a strategic resource, central to the core business of health care, or is IT a supporting player, important for conducting business but ultimately adding only incremental value? Differing answers to those questions have led to two prevalent views of the chief information officer:

- The CIO as "application provider"—similar to the IS director's position. Organizations with this view regard the CIO as a supporter of the organization, primarily focused on enabling operations and managing "technology."
- The CIO as "strategic contributor"—the CIO, as general manager and leader, is expected to offer relevant business contributions, as well as to both lead and support organizational success.

Matching the Executive and the Organization

As delivery systems form, grow, and mature, they require different skills and management focus on the part of the chief information officer. At each stage, the true value and potential possible from information technology is dependent on the type of organization, the complexity of its structure, the stage of its organizational development, and the makeup of the executive management team. Table 5.1 describes the basic role of the CIO at various stages of delivery system growth and development.

Table 5.1. The Role of the Chief Information Officer

Organization State[a]	Organization Focus	Role of the Chief Information Officer
Conceptual	New organization; focus on evaluating viability and making basic organizational structure decisions	*Ambassador and visualizer:* primary role is to open doors, develop relationships within and outside the organization to support use of IT, and establish expectations of and for the IT function.
Embryonic	Established basic structure; focus on building core infrastructure	*Operator:* primary role is to develop structure where little or none exists and to solve problems.
Maintenance	Established core infrastructure; focus on day-to-day operations	*Preserver:* primary role is to keep operations running smoothly and to manage incremental change.
Breakthrough	Fully operational organization; focus on change or adapting to new markets or requirements (not every organization enters this phase)	*Visionary:* primary role is to keep the organization moving, to build and sustain viability, and to head in new directions through IT use.

[a]Conceptual organizations, because they lack sunk investment in infrastructure, are typically freer to act as breakthrough organizations.

CIO Responsibilities

Whether given the title of CIO or IS director, this individual is responsible for oversight and leadership of the information technology function in the health care organization. In most organizations, this includes leading efforts to plan and manage information as an organizational resource, as well as establishing and maintaining operational order and core systems.

The CIO may or may not have a technical background; there are any number of successful individuals performing the CIO function with a management-level understanding of IT rather than a deeply technical one. The general roles and responsibilities that should be filled by the top IT executive include some combination of the following:

- Executive team membership, with leadership, financial, strategic, and operational responsibilities
- Enterprisewide (IDS) information systems policy setting and management, either through line control with affiliated facilities or entities (such as home health, managed care, management services organizations, and physician-hospital organizations)
- IS department managers as direct reports or as a corporate-level facilitator of IS planning and management
- Development of, facilitation of, and consultation with the organizational IT governance body
- Information technology planning and development, including future trend analysis and forecasting, technology scanning and adaptation analysis, capital allocations and budgeting, and when applicable, alpha or beta site development responsibilities
- Regulatory compliance management, including Joint Commission on Accreditation of Healthcare Organizations (JCAHO) information management and Health Insurance Portability and Accountability Act (HIPAA) regulatory mandates

- External relationship management, including (but not limited to) IT vendors, outsourcers, systems integrators, consultants, and others involved in the development or support of IT goals and systems

- Internal relationship management, developing and sustaining IT satisfaction levels of executive peers and organizational end users

- Systems and technology implementation and operations (in an oversight role)

- Telecommunications and network implementation and operations (in an oversight role)

- Management education (of IT's relevance to business and medical service objectives, including the potentials of new and emerging technologies)

- General management oversight (may hold responsibility for other groups within the organization, such as medical records, business office, decision support, or management engineering—any function that deals routinely with large amounts of data and information)

In recognition of the complexity of the CIO role, some health care organizations are committing to additional IS-related executive positions, some of which are discussed in the next section.

Emerging Executive Roles

The breathtaking scope of information technology and the widely divergent demands placed on the chief information officer are leading some organizations to split the CIO role into parts. Other executives sometimes found in health care organizations today include the chief technology officer (CTO), the chief knowledge officer (CKO), and the chief medical information officer (CMIO).

The chief technology officer is typically responsible for managing technical operations and maintenance, particularly of the foundation technologies of the organization (for example, networks, hardware, telecommunications and Internet-intranet-extranet). Often the second in command, the CTO reports directly to the CIO. The chief knowledge officer (CKO) is responsible for creating tools to manage corporate "knowledge" (versus static data or information).

In an effort to increase the participation of physicians in planning and using technology, a growing number of health care organizations are creating the paid position of chief medical information officer (typically held by a physician). The CMIO is most commonly responsible for acting as a liaison between the IS department and affiliated clinical staff, working to train and educate physicians about IT, as well as to involve them in the planning and selection of applications for their use.

Though still not very common, these new and emerging executive positions reflect the increasing acknowledgment of the difficulty of the CIO function. In coming years, the CIO role will continue to shift and evolve as health care organizations adopt management models in line with changing organizational goals and expectations.

Management Challenges

Whatever the composition of the management team, each health care IS department must navigate a number of common challenges that relate primarily to organizational expectations, culture, and operational structure: managing changing relationships, setting consistent and realistic expectations, engaging the executive team, aligning departmental and organizational structures, and recruiting and retaining key staff and leaders.

Managing Changing Relationships. More than ever before, developing and maintaining workable partnerships with internal and external constituencies is critical to IS survival. Yet those relationships are facing daily changes. New outsourcing models, the changing technical requirements of Internet technologies, and the growing involvement of health care organizations with emerging technologies are requiring more intimate connections between IS and external technology suppliers. Concurrently, internal health care organization mandates to "be strategic," increased management decentralization, and the involvement of end users in IS planning and decision making all require IS to solidify internal relationships.

Setting Consistent and Realistic Expectations. More than one CIO's tenure has been cut short by an inability to manage organizational expectations for information technology. The realities of conflicting organizational priorities, capital budget competition, existing IT competency (or lack thereof), and IT staff size and capabilities make it literally impossible to achieve unlimited goals relating to technology. Executives who cannot clearly communicate the limits of what can be accomplished and involve the organization in priority setting, no matter how talented, will be viewed as less than competent. At the same time, those who consistently set low expectations, whether or not they deliver on them, undermine their credibility as part of the organizational executive team. Walking a balance between these two extremes requires thoughtfulness, clear and well-developed management communication skills, and a core understanding of how IT can support organizational mission.

Engaging the Executive Team. The perception of information technology in the organization begins with the executive office suite. Engaging the *entire* executive team in the potential and actual benefits of information technology is an essential skill for a CIO. At every organizational development stage, the CIO is part educator; discussions sponsored and led by the CIO and presentations about the relevance of technology raise awareness of the importance of IT. The focus of these presentations *must match the technical interest and knowledge of the executive audience,* or they will be counterproductive. Strong and consistent governance (also discussed later in this chapter) is another mechanism through which the CIO can involve organizational executives in information technology.

Aligning Departmental and Organizational Structures. The operational and functional structure of the IS department must be consistent with the expectations, culture, and structure of the larger health care organization. Specific staffing models and approaches (discussed later in this chapter) must adequately support the business and medical service requirements of the health care organization, including both existing and planned information technology infrastructures.

Recruiting and Retaining Key Staff and Leaders. Today's marketplace does not support the view of IT staff as "disposable"; in fact, just the opposite. With so many emerging technologies being planned and deployed, there are simply not enough competent and experienced technical staff to go around. Complicating matters, as formerly director-level staff members have moved into the upper ranks of executives, the concomitant shifting of analyst and technical staff into supervisor and manager positions has stretched many organizations thin.

Competition for information technology talent (at the executive and staff levels) is especially fierce, with organizations across a spectrum of industries vying for a finite pool of qualified candidates. Even within health care, provider organizations must compete for key talent not only with one another but also with systems integrators, IT vendors, and consulting firms (many of which are able to offer more appealing compensation packages).

In managing this issue, many health care organizations habitually promote internal staff to available positions. The success of these promotions can be strongly influenced by existing cultural perceptions and relationships; mentoring these individuals and establishing internal development programs to overcome gaps or deficiencies is crucially important. (Unfortunately, strong technical managers do not always make effective chief information officers, and strong business managers do not always have enough technical understanding to succeed; internal staff education and professional development are therefore critical organizational responsibilities.)

OVERSIGHT AND GOVERNANCE

The most effective CIOs are supported by a strong, participatory, and clearly defined oversight and governance function. As a management tool, governance provides a structured mechanism for executives and users to participate in the planning, execution, and oversight of information technology at the organization. Particularly in an integrated delivery system environment, strong governance is required to ensure organizational continuity and focus on a shared IT vision.

Governance Structure and Models

The governance function for information technology should consist primarily of a committee led by a key non-CIO organizational executive (preferably the chief executive officer). This committee should have representation from all critical organizations, departments, and units, including key user and clinical constituencies. It should have clearly defined roles and expectations (individuals may have limited exposure to IT, and all participants will have competing time demands). And it must meet regularly.

Organizations may adopt either centralized or distributed approaches to IT governance. *Centralized* governance committees serve as the default decision-making and planning body for all IT-related decisions. Only decisions specifically excluded from oversight should be made elsewhere (an example might be deciding on the standard desktop hardware configuration for end users). Organizations taking the *decentralized* approach make the governance committee responsible for only the specific decision areas specifically chartered to them (such as strategic direction setting or enterprise systems planning). Decentralized governance is more common for larger health care organizations and multiregion integrated delivery systems.

In either approach, many organizations now create project-specific governance committees for key strategic or emerging technology projects (such as the planning and implementation of an enterprisewide electronic medical record or planning a postmerger IS structure). This allows a closer focus on a specific critical project than a single committee structure might allow.

Governance Responsibilities

Governance committees should always have clearly focused responsibilities for specific activities. Whereas operational functions (systems implementation, network and data center operations) can be monitored in an oversight role, the cross-departmental, organizational, and user nature of the committee will best serve at the strategy and direction level.

Typical responsibilities include the following:

- Defining the appropriate relationship between corporate and medical strategies, information technology, and IT investment and return expectations
- Setting priorities and allocating resources
- Providing feedback and strategic direction against corporate philosophy and approach to the CIO
- Overseeing IS department progress toward goals and initiating corrective action if projects, programs, or executives deviate from agreed parameters
- Setting organizational standards for data sharing, security, privacy, and confidentiality

The governance committee offers the CIO powerful support in managing new, unexpected, or complex situational challenges. Some of the circumstances that can be managed more effectively using governance support are detailed in Table 5.2.

Working in concert, the CIO and the governance committee can maintain a focused and consistent vision and application of standards to information technology at the health care organization.

THE INFORMATION SYSTEMS DEPARTMENT AND OPERATIONS

The structure of the IS department can take many forms, depending on the size and complexity of the health care organization, the organization's focus, and its expectations from information technology. "Form follows function" is certainly a truism applicable to health care IS departments; selecting a management structure that mirrors the functions the department provides and the overall relationships to affiliated organizations establishes a firm foundation for success.

Table 5.2. Situational Governance

Organizational Challenge	Governance Role or Approach
Keeping physicians close to the organization	• Common IT initiatives (such as e-commerce and clinical IT) that require close planning and oversight • Risk identification and management
Joint venture and alliance communication	• Extraorganizational data-sharing standards and agreement
IT vision and planning	• Prioritization and resource allocation • Continuity and long-term organizational focus • Defining the appropriate relationship between corporate strategy, information systems, and technology and establishing investment expectations
Emerging IT and special projects	• Managing added risk • Cross-organizational exposure and complexity • Higher visibility; initiating corrective action if projects, programs, or executives deviate from established parameters
Times of transition (merger, acquisition, rapid growth)	• Consensus building • Building a shared vision for the future • Focus and oversight; controlling investments, and keeping the organization "on track"

Organizational Structures

Information systems departments and operations can assume many structural variations. As noted in Chapter Three, IDS formation and regional and corporate structures and strategies are driving a diverse and changing mix of centralized, decentralized, and distributed IT approaches and management functions. The size and complexity of the health care organization drive many of these decisions.

Less complex organizations may choose to divide information services into three or four functional units, each with assigned IT-related responsibilities (see Exhibit 5.1).

Larger or more complex organizations often adopt different models, designed for the cross-facility, cross-organizational business structures they must support. One increasingly common approach to structuring IDS information systems operations is the formation of a centralized service organization to hold responsibility for specific information technology areas, with all other functions being managed directly at the individual facility or region level.

Key to success with this approach is identifying which specific systems and functions are most logically and cost-effectively managed at a central level, balanced against individual facility need and desire for autonomy and control. Exhibit 5.2 shows one example of how a central service organization's responsibilities might be delineated, with unassigned responsibilities managed at the individual entity or facility level.

Key Functions and Responsibilities

Large or small, the IS department is typically responsible for a number of key functions within the health care organization. Critical responsibilities that must be filled at some level of the IS departmental structure include these:

- Overall department coordination, planning, and management
- Operations, including network, Internet-intranet-extranet systems, telecommunication systems management, database management, disaster planning, and security control

Exhibit 5.1. Small Delivery Systems

Planning Unit

- Strategy

- Development of technical standards, investment criteria, financial requirements and policies, and ROI expectations and guidelines

- Postimplementation ROI analysis

- Customer satisfaction

- Leadership of "strategic" (emerging technology) projects

Operations Unit

- Classic data-processing functions—hardware and application software

- Help desk, user support

- Computer operations—data center, backups, reports

- Possible telecommunications responsibility

Technical Support Unit

- Hardware support and maintenance

- Cabling plans and changes

- Network management (including Internet access, intranet, local and wide area networks)

Systems Unit

- Selection, implementation, development, or customization of application solutions

- Systems maintenance

- Systems documentation

- User group, end user training

Note: Organizations may have one, several, or all of the units described.

Exhibit 5.2. Sample Central Service Organization Structure and Responsibilities

Technical Services

- Network administration and planning
- Telecommunications
- Data center operations
- End user support (help desk)

Provider Services

- Helping physicians and caregivers access and use available IT effectively

Data Integration

- Planning and responding to cross-organizational data sharing and security requirements (data warehousing, interface engines, Internet-intranet-extranet systems, e-commerce, consumer outreach)

Systems Planning and Integration

- Coordinating and managing core applications that are standardized across the health system
- Planning and managing emerging technology projects with high potential returns, risk, or visibility

---

- Planning (including strategic planning), new technology evaluation, and intra-IDS and inter-IDS project development
- Systems development and implementation, including new systems selection and cost specification, project planning and management, internal application development, and management report development
- Systems maintenance, including application support and maintenance of custom or vendor-supplied software where appropriate

- User support, including help desk management, user manual updates, user group coordination, and user training.

Some of these functions are consistently undermanaged or overlooked by provider organizations—in some cases because responsibility for the area is relatively new, in others because the impact of the activity is not fully understood by the department.

Internet and Electronic Commerce Initiative Management

With the level of excitement and initiative being applied to Internet and electronic commerce projects, the stark reality that emerges is this: *if you don't build it, the end users will.* The revolutionary changes of Internet technology go well beyond the walls of the IS department. Even technology neophytes have gained some level of conceptual understanding of what may be possible to achieve via the World Wide Web.

Health care IS departments that don't funnel and control this energy will ultimately be controlled by it. Today, some organizations struggle even to produce a simple list of Internet-related initiatives in operation with the health system. Putting even simple management controls around such initiatives, such as creating a centralized management office to oversee and coordinate organizational efforts, is an important first step toward more effective oversight. Incorporating Internet technology as a separate planning track (the emerging technology component of the long-range plan, discussed in Chapter Four) is another.

Information Security and Confidentiality

All too often, information security and confidentiality emerge as an afterthought of systems management or after a highly visible security violation. The issues around protecting the integrity and confidentiality of data—particularly patient data—will continue to gain prominence as the requirements of HIPAA are defined, enacted, implemented, and enforced.

Every health care organization should establish a clear mandate to develop and maintain standards and policies that restrict the access of information in accordance with job responsibility and organizational access. A comprehensive approach to this concern has three components: policy setting, technical implementation, and end user education.

Policy Setting. Normally set and approved by the IS governance function, the organizational security policy should at a minimum deal with global issues of data standards, collection, and management, as well as any extra-organizational data sharing.

When setting policies, the governance committee should consider the unique risks the health care organization faces in terms of protecting patient data. Large amounts of computerized clinical patient data, and transmission of data across the Internet are two common risk factors health care organizations must deal with. An additional risk relates to data that are being transmitted across vendor networks. A number of companies are attempting to contractually gain ownership or use rights to patient data traversing their networks. Others are claiming sole intellectual property rights to co-developed or customized application software. Health care organizations must be cautious in granting these privileges.

Technical Implementation. A wide range of security systems and technologies are commercially available, and most application systems come with some built-in controls. The challenge for IS is to determine the combination of technologies that offers adequate protection at a cost-effective price. Some of these systems offer *user identification and access management tools*—technologies that clearly identify end users and manage the level and extent of system and data access they receive—for example, user passwords, biometric (fingerprint, retinal scan) systems, audit logs, and user-defined "roles" and privileges. Other systems offer *connectivity, data exchange, and commerce tools*—technologies that protect data from being inappropriately accessed by remote or unintended recipients. Examples include callback systems that dial only preapproved remote access numbers, firewalls, and public key infrastructure encryption.

End User Education. Although computerized data security is an articulated responsibility of the IS department, any approach, to be successful, must be a collaborative effort involving both policy-setting and operational groups within the organization. It is impossible to implement a set of security policies without the complete agreement and support of the users who will be affected. If the user population does not feel a sense of ownership and responsibility for securing data and conforming to policies, those policies will inevitably fail.

Disaster Planning

Every year, a number of health care organizations encounter crisis situations brought on by natural or other disasters. In these instances, providers may face a disruption in information services (through power failure, forced evacuation, or building damage). Regional trauma centers and other institutions with high-volume emergency centers are particularly vulnerable during times of natural disaster, and disaster planning is critical if these institutions are to provide needed levels of health care during a crisis.

Development of the organizationwide disaster plan should include an IS component. Moreover, IS management should identify potential risks to the systems and develop procedures—in consultation with senior management—to ensure system availability during a disaster recovery period.

There are many levels of disaster recovery, from simple downed systems that are addressable by operations management to larger-scale disasters that require the relocation of IT services, where all affected staff need to understand their role thoroughly. Disaster planning proves a difficult task for many organizations. No one enjoys thinking about fires, floods, bombings, or earthquakes. In addition, ignoring or underfunding disaster-response capabilities is easy to do when the sun is shining and the earth is still. The consequences of not planning (lost lives, damaged property, interrupted business, failure in the eyes of the community) are potentially overwhelming.

MEASURING UP: IS DEPARTMENT BEST PRACTICES

The ultimate success of the IS executive and department in an organization is dependent on many management, cultural, and technological factors, making "best practices" difficult to define. These organizations share a commitment to quality assurance tools, technology proficiency, and clearly structured management and oversight. Structures, models, and approaches take many forms—but "best practice" IS departments have many similarities.

Just as organizations at different stages need different characteristics in their chief information officer, they need different characteristics in their IS department. True success can only be defined by the individual health care organization. In forming that definition, there are a number of obvious questions:

- What are our organizational needs and expectations relating to IT? Are they being adequately served?

- For the amount of money being spent, are we receiving value?

- Is the IS function being managed according to basic accepted management principles?

Even within a health care organization, different perceptions of what constitutes success will inevitably exist. The chief financial officer's definition may relate to adherence to budgets, whereas physicians' definitions may relate to the presence or absence of automated clinical support tools (such as results reports or electronic medical records). The vice president for human resources may look at staff salaries and turnover; the admitting office staff, at application availability, functionality, ease of use, and help desk service. In assessing the quality of the IS function, it is necessary to incorporate all of these valid viewpoints and examine operational, strategic, and political competencies.

Operational Competencies

Operational competencies relate to the day-to-day management and effectiveness of the department. Maintaining key competencies ensures department efficiency.

Systems are available and response time is within acceptable parameters. Despite the new focus on information technology as a strategic resource, successful departments never neglect the basics—information systems should be available, with little or no "surprise" downtime. The credibility of the department in larger, more strategic projects can be critically undermined if it fails to manage the existing systems and infrastructure in a competent manner.

The help desk function is effective. Staff members keep open communication with users about pending issues; there are clear problem resolution and escalation procedures; basic statistics about calls and issues are tracked and reported.

Vendor relationships are clearly and proactively managed. Maintenance contracts and responsibilities are clear and auditable. Issue severity and escalation policies are consistent and adhered to.

Projects are competently managed. Projects are managed to reasonable deadlines, within established budget parameters. Department management knows how many projects are open at any particular time.

System and staff outsourcing is appropriately evaluated and managed. New outsourcing models, such as those offered by application service providers, judiciously adopted, can reduce operating and staff costs as well as provide organizations access to new and emerging technologies that might otherwise be out of reach. However, as attractive as these models appear, core competencies in IT planning as well as management accountability should *never* be removed from the health care organization itself.

Executive and staff turnover is at or below industry standards. New management personnel have to invest sometimes significant amounts of time building relationships with department staff, organizational end users, and vendor personnel.

Strategic Competencies

Strategic competencies describe the value that information technology provides to the larger health care organization. The following circumstances are characteristic of success in this area.

Major IS areas of responsibility are tied directly to business or medical services. The IS department must always be able to articulate how it contributes to the overall health and efficiency of the organization. *This competency is central to IS department success.* If the CIO cannot document that IS has a direct, measurable impact on the core business of the health care organization—delivering, financing, or managing health care—he or she risks being marginalized, cut out of organizational decisions, or fired.

Effective IS departments conduct clear and proactive technology planning, involving key executives and linking IT as closely as possible with the larger organizational business plan or subsidiary business plans. The most effective IT planning efforts actually uncover new organizational possibilities (for example, new advances in data mining technology bringing to light new service demand potential). While this effort may be complicated if the organization has no strategic business plan, every attempt should be made to align IT goals and strategies with those of the larger organization.

Return-on-investment measurement and continuous quality improvement are realities. Follow-up studies, both qualitative and quantitative, are conducted for new technologies. Central project issues are reviewed, including team structure and composition, project organizational structure, and issue resolution techniques, with learning experiences incorporated into future projects. The IS function takes the lead in exploring and using new technology, even acting as a technology transfer agent between organizational functions and departments.

Political Competencies

Political competencies relate to how the IS function is positioned within the larger organization. Is IS purely a line function, or does the department (and the CIO) participate at the executive management level? Success in this area can be characterized in the following ways.

Clinicians, end users, and executives have clear and realistic expectations. Setting appropriate expectations for information systems in this fast-paced marketplace is another key challenge for IT executives. The past decade of experience with health care IT has consistently shown the value and influence of "IS champions"—executives or clinicians willing to get involved directly in the IS planning and use processes. Effective IS management demands widespread and direct involvement of non-IS constituencies—as governance committee members, educational session participants, alpha and beta site test subjects, and end users.

In particular, as clinical information technology continues to develop over the next decade, the intimate involvement of physicians and other clinical staff in IS department planning and education should correspondingly grow.

Customer perception and satisfaction are measured and found to be high. The level of satisfaction that organizational customers feel with information technology, and with the IS department, is almost always directly correlated with the extent of end user education and involvement. However, it is important that the IS department periodically conduct formal reviews of customer satisfaction. In conducting such reviews, IS executives and staff will not only gain valuable feedback on their own performance in supporting organization needs but also gain insight into the ways that end users access technologies and ways to improve both the level and quality of that access.

The department has regular and structured approaches to soliciting end user and executive involvement and IS education. Even the most functional and advanced technology can fail if it does not meet what users see as their critical needs or if users are not aware of its full potential. To avoid these situations, the IS department should vigorously pursue the involvement and participation of all key user constituencies in IS activities and decisions.

The IS department should develop and maintain a rigorous training program for new users as well as "refresher" training for continuing users. With the current pace of change in technology, application systems, in particular, can look very different after only a year or two, with new and enhanced features and functionalities as well as user access tools. By placing a continued emphasis on training, the IS department can ensure that users are aware of the most current and beneficial ways to use technology.

Outside Influences

However positive the internal indicators may be, there are a number of external factors that can influence the effectiveness of an IS function.

Vendor Staffing Issues. Just as provider organizations do, technology suppliers, software developers, outsourcers, and application service providers can struggle when staff or management turnover is high or uncontrolled. A number of provider organizations have found themselves in the position of having internal staff with more comprehensive system knowledge than the staff of the vendor organization. Under normal circumstances, this may not make much of an impact. But in cases where the health care organization desires a number of customizations or complicated adaptations, the vendor organization product is not yet fully developed, or the vendor holds responsibility for operations, support, or systems integration, vendor staffing problems can have a negative impact on IS department productivity and workflow.

The "Dot-Com" Phenomenon. The tremendous hype and stock variability of "dot-com" companies has many executives paying closer note to these information technology investments than to other organizational vendors. In some cases, the excitement around these vendors leads to greater focus on them than on companies providing software, services, or support for the health care organization's core business processes.

The business failure or significant redirection of a core system vendor—such as the hospital information system used at one or more of the IDS hospitals—is far more likely to have a detrimental and long-term affect than the failure of the vendor with whom the IDS is conducting a small-scale wireless technology beta test.

SUMMARY

Successful information systems management requires competent and dedicated leadership and staff as well as a management structure that optimizes the use and maintenance of technology within a given organization. As the health care organization evolves in response to financial, clinical, and business issues and trends, so must the information services department. This is particularly true during periods of rapid consolidation and market change, characterized by mergers, acquisitions, and joint ventures.

The role of information technology and the IS department in health care organizations has changed considerably over the past several years and will continue to evolve. The potential and the challenge of information technology will grow as developers create new and more ingenious applications for health care, and providers continue to develop management skill in adopting and exploiting new capabilities. Strategic vision, effective IT management, and planning competencies will keep information technology high on the list of competitive differentiators and critical support systems far into the future.

Appendix: Technology Concepts

I t is undeniable that the chief executive officer plays a critical enabling role in the successful planning and use of information technology at the health care organization. Clearly, the CEO must understand the business potential and the financial ramifications of using (or not using) health care IT. Exactly how much, though, does the CEO need to know about the technology itself?

Some executives enthusiastically submerge themselves in the workings of IT, studying network topologies, RAM, DRAM, SDRAM, broadband speeds, and Internet communication protocols. Others avoid technical subjects as completely as possible, paying attention only when financial decisions are submitted for review and approval or when related organizational crises or regulatory mandates require executive attention. Both approaches are problematic. The overenthusiastic executive risks getting mired in technical detail and micromanagement, losing sight of broader business requirements; the avoidant leader risks losing technology-enabled or -driven opportunities by not understanding fully how to balance the bottom-line costs against the optimal technology benefit.

This appendix offers a basic review of information technology concepts and terminology with which the CEO should have at least a passing acquaintance.

WHAT DOES A CHIEF EXECUTIVE NEED TO KNOW?

Controlling information technology is a basic executive responsibility, much like establishing effective personnel policies, ensuring healthy cash flows, and maintaining solid departmental operations. The appropriate level of executive knowledge is no higher or lower than that needed to carry out any other responsibility.

In short, all chief executives need what can be characterized as a good "walking-around" knowledge of information technology. With this strong overall understanding of the systems field, the executive can develop a high level of confidence in dealing with systems issues and the ability to sense when someone is giving incomplete or inaccurate information (without necessarily knowing precisely what is wrong with the presentation or what the correct answers are).

A BASIC INTRODUCTION

A *computer* is a digital or electronic machine that carries out logic activities, computations, data manipulation, and text editing under the direction of a set of instructions called a *program*. Computers are generalists—that is, they are machines that were not designed for a specific purpose. The computer equipment that handles financial data processing or moves information between nursing stations and ancillary departments is a general-purpose machine. With different programs, it could be running the checkout terminals at a supermarket or the financial affairs of the local bank.

Some computers, however, are designed for a specific purpose. These truly programmable machines are used to control an airplane, monitor a car engine, direct the activities of a machine tool, or control and monitor laboratory instruments or radiology equipment in a hospital. In general, special-purpose computers are more efficient in carrying out the specific tasks for which they were designed. Whether product designers use general- or special-purpose computers in a given product or system is primarily a matter of economics. (Both kinds are used in health care organizations.)

Hardware and Peripherals

Computer *hardware* (equipment) can be purchased in many forms. However, as technology has developed, the boundaries and differences between

PCs, minicomputers, superminicomputers, and mainframes have blurred. Many of today's personal computers have far more processing power than early mainframe computers. As technological advances allow the basic circuitry of computers to become smaller, more reliable, and less expensive, the capabilities of smaller computers have increased significantly.

To perform tasks, computer hardware must be combined with two additional elements: more machines (called *peripherals*) and *software* (instructions) to tell all of the machines what to do. Taken together, a computer (or computer network) plus peripherals plus software equals a computer system. It is the computer *system* that actually performs tasks and generates information.

Peripherals fall into three categories:

- *Input devices,* which move information into the computer, where it may be processed, passed along to an output device, or stored in memory

- *Output devices,* which take information from the computer in some type of electronic code, convert it into words or numbers, and present it

- *Memory storage devices,* which provide long-term storage of coded information

Software is the most important part of information technology (at least to the user). A computer needs two types of software: *systems* software and *application* software. Computer software is available in a number of languages and maintained in a number of ways to keep it up-to-date.

Systems software is what the computer uses to control its own internal operations—the coming and going of data, the allocation of space in main memory, the logging of activities, and so on. The major component of a computer's system software is called the *operating system*. This is almost always purchased at the same time as the computer hardware.

Besides an operating system, the information systems department may want additional internal software to help optimize computer effectiveness. Examples of such software include a security system to control access, an analyzer to monitor how much main memory is being used and by whom, and various tools for enhancing system efficiency. Any piece of systems software that is not part of the operating system is generally referred to as a *system utility.*

Databases

As providers continue to integrate health care services, the ability to store, manipulate, and analyze large data sets is increasingly important. Longitudinal cost and outcome studies mandate access to a large body of data often collected at different times and at separate points of care. Modern *database technology* offers relational capabilities and open, standardized database access tools such as Structured Query Language (SQL), Open Database Connectivity (ODBC), and Java Database Connectivity (JDBC).

These tools have allowed health care providers to access data at the point in the network where the data can offer the greatest value. *Data repositories,* which collect, filter, and normalize information from other information systems, permit flexible, user-defined data requests and formatting.

TELECOMMUNICATIONS AND NETWORKING

Discussions about *telecommunications* have historically focused on telephone systems; today, this area has broadened to encompass a much broader set of technologies. Modern telephone circuitry carries digital signals, which can be used to transmit voice signals, computer signals, or even digitized video signals (for example, digitized EKG tracings or the output of a digital radiography unit). Technologies that use telecommunications circuitry include both voice (telephone) and data (computer systems) connections.

All signals transmitted over telecommunications lines have a *bandwidth,* a size measurement proportional to the amount of data transmitted or received over time. As the world becomes increasingly interconnected via telephone, cellular phone, and private and public computer networks, the amount of bandwidth required has increased dramatically. Connectivity technologies, including *digital subscriber line* (DSL), are in growing demand among individuals and organizations who seek to keep connection and transmission speeds high.

Networks

Networking is tying together a group of computers and associated peripherals via a common communications line, storing common applications and data on a single central computer (a *server*). When a network serves a small geographical area, it is referred to as a *local area network* (LAN). In much the same way that cabling for telephones and electrical power is laid through a given area so that phones and electrical devices can be moved around at will and plugged in to wall jacks as needed, computer network cabling is also prelaid to accommodate change and growth.

Over larger geographical areas, organizations may develop *wide area networks* (WANs), connecting end users' computers to network devices (*servers, controllers, managers*) that serve as "traffic cops" for data and system access. Networks can have other uses besides tying together data system devices. Modern network technology allows an organization to use common wiring and connectivity for voice, data, video, and telemetry applications.

Data Security

There are a number of tools in use today that are designed to protect the security and confidentiality of data traveling over public and private networks. A *digital certificate* is one of several electronic means used to secure Internet-based transactions. Issued by a *certificate authority,* a digital certificate contains enough information to authenticate the identity of a person or organization sending or receiving data over the Internet. Digital certificates are increasingly being used in health care, as health care providers and payers continue to expand the amount of business and communications conducted over the Internet.

Encryption is another tool used to secure data being transmitted electronically. Encrypted data are converted from their original form into a form that cannot be understood except by the intended recipient of the data, who has possession of an algorithm that will unscramble the data.

Firewalls are electronic programs that provide an electronic barrier between an organization's internal, private data and operations and the outside world. As requests for data access are received by the firewall, the program examines the appropriateness of the request, for example: Is this request originating from an internal computer or one outside the organization? Can this user be authenticated, and if so, does this user have privileges allowing access to the data the user wants to see?

Viruses are electronic programs that attach to computer files, changing their nature in some way. Some viruses are minor, causing little or no damage; others can corrupt computer hard drives or networks, shutting them down, causing data loss, business stoppage, or other serious events. Viruses can infect executable program files, e-mail systems, or simple data (word processing or spreadsheet) files. Protecting systems from viruses requires a combination of corporate policies, such as restrictions on what types and originators people can accept electronic files from, and technical tools, such as *antivirus software,* that checks new files against a list of known viruses.

Systems Integration and Interfaces

Technically speaking, an *integrated system* (or *consolidated system*) is one in which all data from various applications and systems are collected by the system and reside in a single database, accessible via all system terminals. Theoretically, it is possible to build a single, totally integrated system that meets all of a health system's needs. Often there are several systems, each with its own database, connected to one another by specialized software called *interfaces.* The main purpose of interfaces is to make a system look integrated to the end user. Interfaces are "gateways" that allow systems to interact and appear integrated. And like any other software, interfaces have to be designed, maintained, and upgraded.

Client-Server Architecture

The *client-server* (C/S) structure is one of the most important networking computing concepts of the past decade. It describes the relationship between two or more computers, in which one computer (the client) requests some data or action by the other (the server). A C/S variant called a *three-tier client-server* adds "middleware" between the client and the server to conduct specific predetermined business applications. With host-centered computing, such activities as data processing, storage, and retrieval are concentrated on one central mainframe or minicomputer, with "dumb" (nonprocessing) terminals presenting data to end users. Client-server architecture allows the distribution of data processing, storage, retrieval, and presentation across multiple powerful servers, data repositories, and end user PCs or workstations.

Barriers to C/S architecture have reduced the speed with which health care providers are adopting this systems approach. Many health care providers attempting to implement C/S have seen their costs increase; others have found the technical complexity difficult to manage. Typical C/S configurations contain multiple hardware platforms, networks (cables, routers, protocols), operating systems, databases, and development software and middleware tools. Nevertheless, C/S potential in health care remains high, with ROI potential for electronic medical and health records, clinical data repositories, imaging, and decision support applications.

THE INTERNET AND RELATED TECHNOLOGIES

A network of networks, the *Internet* is a worldwide system of computers and computer networks. Publicly accessible to anyone with access to a computer and an *Internet service provider* (ISP), a company providing access to the Internet over its own communication lines, the Internet has revolutionized computing as we know it. In health care, many organizations have taken advantage of the accessibility of the Internet by creating and maintaining *Web sites,* collections of organization-specific data that any Internet user can access. The most common Internet application in use is *electronic mail,* or *e-mail,* a nearly instantaneous form of electronic communication.

Two increasingly common related technologies are *intranets* and *extranets*. These are networks that use or connect to the Internet but restrict data access to a limited field of participants. Intranets are normally accessible only by users within a particular enterprise, while extranets use a combination of intranet and Internet technology to share on a secure basis some amount of an enterprise's private data with outside parties (such as patients, trading partners, or vendors).

Glossary

affiliation IDS model An integrated delivery system structure through which providers form a loose confederation, focusing on mutually beneficial collaboration while commonly retaining separate management and operations.

alpha site The first place where new software is tested in a true operational environment. Not all technology vendors use this term; some refer to all test organizations as *beta sites.*

American National Standards Institute (ANSI) A national organization that acts as a clearinghouse for voluntary standards in a variety of industries, including health care.

ancillary department systems Technologies that manage activities internal to individual hospital departments, such as laboratory, radiology, pharmacy, and the operating room.

application service provider (ASP) A company providing remote access to and administration of application software (such as a physician practice management system), ordinarily responsible for system installation, maintenance, and upgrades, as well as for providing necessary hardware and network security.

application software A computer program that carries out a specific business or personal task, such as registering a patient, processing an order, or producing a bill.

artificial intelligence (AI) A knowledge-based computer capability in which the computer either actually mimics the thought process of a human being or in some way generates new knowledge. See also *expert system.*

benchmarking See *best practices.*

best practices An IT management tool, also called *benchmarking,* in which the plans and activities of outside organizations successfully using a technology are studied for possible adoption or modification. Also sometimes referred to as *systems use audits.*

beta site The client facility where new software is tested once alpha site testing has been completed. Beta testing focuses on the ability of the vendor to install and support software without the assistance of the software designers. Some vendors do not differentiate between alpha and beta site testing.

bundled Including hardware, software, and implementation services for a set price, leaving the buyer with fewer choices regarding components and levels of service than if the supplier's wares were unbundled.

Business to Technology Alignment methodology A way of viewing the systems life cycle that focuses on identifying and exploiting the interdependencies between business practices and technology potential.

capitated reimbursement A guaranteed monthly payment to providers of a fixed sum for each individual whose health care needs are covered. The fixed fee is paid regardless of the intensity and level of services provided.

central service organization An organization that assumes responsibility for a particular set of functions for associated IDS provider organizations. These may include information systems, managed care contracting, centralized business or financial processing, or materials management.

chief information officer (CIO) Executive responsible for strategic and operational direction of information systems. Not all facilities include this position; however, the responsibilities related to IT must still be performed.

chief knowledge officer (CKO)   Executive responsible for creating tools and processes to manage corporate "knowledge" (as differentiated from static data or information).

chief medical information officer (CMIO)   Executive (typically a physician) who acts as a liaison between the information services department and organizational clinical staff. The CMIO works closely with physicians and other caregivers to involve them in the planning and use of IT at the organization.

chief technology officer (CTO)   Executive responsible for managing technical operations and maintenance, especially of foundation technologies (networks, hardware, telecommunications, Internet-intranet-extranet systems, and the like). Also investigates new and emerging technologies for possible adoption.

client-server architecture   A computer data and software interaction configuration that takes advantage of distributed processing power to improve computing speed and end user capacity.

clinical systems   Systems that contribute to the direct management of patient care activities, including order entry, results reporting, acuity classification, and case management.

community health information network (CHIN)   An arrangement between numerous entities (provider, payer, regulatory agency) to share and exchange common data.

computer-telephone integration   A technology that combines the functions and capabilities of telecommunications with computer application systems. Most commonly used to support call centers, nurse triage, continuing education, and consumer-oriented systems.

consumer health systems   Applications directly targeted for use by health care consumers (patients). Functions might include self-triage, self-service appointment scheduling, personal health record maintenance, and other patient-centered activities.

contract issues document (CID)   A document that methodically reviews current and potential issues in connection with a proposed contract.

conversion   The process of shifting from one system to a different system, even if the same vendor supplies both systems.

core competency   A skill or knowledge set closely held by the organization. Organizations with core competencies in information technology plan, select, and implement IT effectively, consistently measuring and achieving clear benefits and return on investment.

core transaction systems   Application systems that provide support for daily operations, including financial, administrative, and clinical functionality.

corporate ownership IDS model   A highly integrated IDS model in which one central corporation controls the individual provider entities, services, and management.

customer relationship management system   Application system that uses computer-telephone integration technology to track, manage, and analyze customer contacts with the organization.

data integration   Connectivity between and across application systems, allowing data input into one system to be accessed from others.

data repository   A data collection and storage tool that can incorporate patient demographic, financial, and clinical information into one physical location, allowing data access and input throughout the enterprise or IDS. Often used synonymously with a *data warehouse.*

data warehouse   A data repository that incorporates strengthened data access and analysis tools.

decision support systems   Applications that allow providers to collect and analyze data in more sophisticated and complex ways. Activities supported include: case mix, budgeting, cost accounting, clinical protocols and pathways, outcomes, and actuarial analysis.

e-commerce   A combination of application systems, advanced technologies, and telecommunications allowing consistent, secure, and reliable communication across often unconnected entities.

e-health   A broad term referring to any electronic exchange of health care data or information across organizations.

electronic data interchange (EDI)   The automated exchange of data and documents in a standardized format. In health care, some common uses of this technology include claims submission and payment, eligibility, and referral authorization.

electronic medical record (EMR)   An application that aggregates patient data from a variety of source systems; advanced EMRs allow access to text, graphics, clinical results, images, voice, and video.

e-mail   A means of sending letters, memos, and other correspondence electronically over a network.

emerging technology   Technology, unproven or untested in the health care industry, offering great potential benefits to organizations willing to accept the associated risks. Some current emerging technologies include workflow, fully functional electronic medical records, telemedical, and telehealth applications.

enterprise system   Applications allowing a single point of access for patient and resource management across a health system or set of connected organizations.

expert system   A system that provides the ability to consolidate a predefined view (from one or more experts) into an application system. The predefined view is then used to process a unique data set against predetermined variables. Used in medical diagnosis, clinical information, and credit and risk assessment systems.

extranet   The part of an enterprise network or intranet that is extended via secure means to specific outside users.

facilities management   An approach to IT management whereby a provider organization enters into a contract with a third party for management or operational IT support. Provider organizations choosing this approach typically maintain their own data center and capital equipment; the facility management firm manages the people and processes relating to IT; compare *outsourcing.*

foundation technology   Technology that allows application systems to communicate more effectively; examples include networking technologies, data integration and interface tools, and computer-telephone integration.

general financial management systems   Technologies that support the basic financial transactions required in the day-to-day operation of a health care enterprise (for example, general ledger, payroll, materials management, human resources).

governance   The structured oversight of information technology at the organizational level. Generally executed through the use of one or more "steering committees" composed of senior executives and a cross-section of organizational constituencies.

hardware   Equipment that runs application software, or peripheral devices (such as printers or computer monitors) used in working with computers.

Health Insurance Portability and Accountability Act (HIPAA)   U.S. law passed in 1996 requiring the adoption of standards for electronic health transactions and requiring specific patient data security and confidentiality measures.

health level seven (HL7)   A data interchange protocol for health care applications that simplifies the ability of different vendor-supplied systems to interconnect. Although not a software program in itself, HL7 requires each software vendor to program HL7 interfaces.

home health systems   Application software designed to support the administrative, financial, and clinical activities relating to home health care.

imaging   The collection, viewing, and manipulation of digital images, whether of a document, a picture, or clinical result data.

information systems (IS)   Application software designed to automate a particular part of the health care process, such as managed care administration, laboratory operations, or patient administration.

information systems steering committee (ISSC)   A governance body, typically responsible for setting and monitoring the organization's overall approach and strategy for information systems and technology management.

information technology (IT)   Technology designed to facilitate process or customer service automation in health care. More than information systems, information technology encompasses application software, operating systems, database and data access systems, telecommunications equipment (networks, telephones), and computer hardware.

information technology planning   The formal process through which an organization assesses its IT status and performance against industry standards, best practices, and current and future expected business requirements and then designs strategies and tactics to target future investment to meet key needs and objectives. Also commonly referred to as *strategic planning* or *long-range planning*.

integrated delivery system (IDS)   A health care provider organization offering support for the majority of care services, incorporating physician groups and focusing on continuity of care management and the management of patient populations. Also called *integrated health delivery network, integrated health network,* or *regional delivery system.*

integrated medical devices   Medical devices that capture, collect, and transmit physiologically oriented data directly into a health care application system. An example of this technology might be a peak flow meter that allows the periodic download of a reading onto a physician's desktop computer.

interface   Specialized software or hardware that permits the passing of information back and forth between two systems. Interfaces are of two types: batch and real-time.

interface engines   A technology that facilitates data transfer and communication between applications that would otherwise be incompatible.

Internet   A worldwide network of networks, allowing public access to anyone with a computer and a service provider.

intranet   A private network for use within an enterprise (and therefore not available to the public).

local area network (LAN)   A communications network linking all system devices within a specific area, such as a department or building floor. A defining characteristic of a LAN, compared with alternative methods of interconnecting a network, is flexibility in adding devices or changing the systems configuration. With a LAN, such activities involve plugging and unplugging devices from preplanned wall jacks and entering instructions into the LAN's file server. With other approaches, adding devices or reconfiguring involves pulling cable.

long-range plan   See *information technology planning.*

managed care systems   Technologies providing support for the multiple and complex contracting arrangements required under managed care reimbursement. Some managed care systems are designed to support health care provider activities relating to managed care; others work with activities of health care payers.

medical management systems   Application systems designed to assist or guide physicians in the process of care provision, working toward optimum outcome at the lowest cost. Common functions include clinical protocols, alerts, reminders, and drug interaction and allergy warnings.

networking and telecommunications   Technologies that allow humans and machines to communicate across geographical distances. Specific technologies include local and wide area networks, telephone systems, EDI, and data interface applications.

office automation   Use of computers and computer networks to accomplish tasks associated with white-collar activities, such as word processing, spreadsheets, e-mail, and message processing.

operations unit The group in the information systems department responsible for supporting the classic data-processing functions of an organization. In most organizations, this unit keeps systems operating twenty-four hours a day, seven days a week.

outsourcing An approach to IT management whereby a provider organization enters into a contract with a third party for management or operational IT support. The provider organization does not maintain control of IT assets and typically does not maintain a data-processing center; compare *facilities management.*

patient administrative and management systems Technologies that deal with the practical, nonclinical aspects of treating patients (such as admissions, registration, scheduling, quality assurance, and utilization review).

physician practice management systems Application software designed to support the financial, administrative, and clinical activities of physician group practice.

pivot opportunity An occasion for an organization to quickly capture and demonstrate value, market share, or product benefits.

planning unit A group often found within the information services department that is responsible for strategy, ROI evaluation, customer satisfaction measurement, and investment standards.

proprietary Limited to use by a single vendor. A proprietary chip is an electronic circuit a hardware maker designed for its own use instead of using "off the shelf" technology.

qualitative benefits Benefits logically inferred to have resulted from the use of a technology but difficult or impossible to tie to the technology directly.

quantitative benefits Measurable financial benefits clearly attributable to the use of a particular technology.

regional delivery IDS model An integrated delivery system structure that emphasizes integration over geographical reach. These IDSs typically work to develop a vertical continuum of services rather than a breadth of horizontal ones.

remote processing   A network configuration in which a data center is removed from the main user areas, as in another building or another country.

replacement market   Marketplace in which potential buyers have some type of system in place, purchasing new systems only to "replace" the old. In the United States market, hospital information systems (such as patient accounting) are considered a replacement market.

request for information (RFI)   A short, high-level document used to collect basic system data as well as vendor marketing literature in some vendor selection projects.

request for proposal (RFP)   A document commonly used by provider organizations during vendor selection projects. Some organizations feel that the RFP, typically binary (containing long series of yes-or-no questions) and extremely detailed, is too cumbersome an instrument for selecting vendors.

research systems   Application systems allowing the collection, consolidation, tracking, management, and analysis of data relating to clinical research efforts (including administrative, financial, and clinical data components).

return on investment (ROI)   The quantitative and qualitative benefits realized by an organization from an investment in information technology. Benefits may or may not be economic; they may also be strategic, positioning an organization for future benefits.

scripted demonstration   A method of reviewing software applications that provides vendors with a specific list of functions or scenarios that they must show. This method can be helpful in bringing to light flaws or gaps in a system's functionality.

security   Tools and techniques used to protect a computer system from unauthorized access.

shared system   A computer configuration in which more than one organization uses the same programs running on the same hardware, all of which are maintained at a central data center. Not to be confused with *remote processing*.

software   Computer programs to control internal computer operations or to carry out the tasks for which an information system is designed. See also *application software* and *systems software.*

source code   Software that is developed in machine language. Also called *object code.*

strategic benefits   Positioning or other benefits that may offer substantial value to the organization but will not necessarily have a direct impact for some time to come.

strategic planning   See *information technology planning.*

systems implementation   The process of incorporating new applications or technologies into a health care organization's operations. Typically a lengthy and detailed process as new data structures, files, and work processes are designed and tested and existing data are converted for use in the new system.

systems integration   Technical and functional programming activities that develop connectivity between legacy systems or new technologies (or both).

systems life cycle   The process through which an investment is planned, selected or developed, implemented, used, and then reevaluated. Activities during the life cycle are geared to optimize and retain the highest rate of return on the investment for the longest period of time.

systems software   A computer program that enables the computer to control its own internal operations, such as controlling the coming and going of data, allocating space in main memory, or logging user activities. Also called *systems program.*

systems unit   Group working in the information systems department to develop, implement, and sometimes customize application software being used by the provider organization. This group is also frequently responsible for end user training.

systems use audit   Activity in which the best practices use of technology is compared to an organization's use, with the goal of increasing the use and value of current information systems.

technical support unit   Group operating within the information systems department that is typically responsible for general PC support and hardware or cabling plans and changes.

telecommunications   See *networking and telecommunications.*

telemedical and telehealth systems   Application systems allowing clinical diagnosis and treatment across geographical distances. These systems typically allow bidirectional transmission of voice, text, and imaging data.

turnkey   Ready for use. Software vendors may provide turnkey products, packages in which all software, hardware, and installation costs are included in a single price.

unbundled   Priced individually. Such "à la carte" pricing allows the buyer of hardware, software, and implementation services to pick and choose which components and levels of support it wants to purchase; compare *bundled.*

vendor selection   Process whereby an organization decides from whom to purchase information systems technology. The vendor selection process quantifies desired organization benefits and objectives and defines technical and operational system requirements.

vendor system proposal (VSP)   A document, issued to potential vendors, that gathers functional, cost, and strategic information about a firm and its products. The VSP is not as detailed as a request for proposal (RFP) but is more detailed than a request for information (RFI).

version   The current edition of a piece of software. Sometimes called *release.*

virtual IDS model   An organizational structure that offers many of the benefits of an integrated delivery system without requiring a formal IDS business or care delivery structure. Group purchasing organizations and many provider-oriented membership organizations can be considered virtual IDSs.

wide area network (WAN)   A communications network linking computers, system devices, and local area networks that are dispersed over a large geographical area, such as a medical center or university campus.

workflow technology   Technology, often integrated into application systems, that supports the daily work processes of end users. Examples include the smart routing of telephone calls and automated work queues for medical management staff.

workforce-enabling technology   Technology that supports education, training, and communication among organizational staff and might include such things as e-mail, groupware and other knowledge management tools, Internet or intranet access, computer-based training, and distance learning.

workstation   An intelligent terminal or personal computer designed for a specific users in a specific industry. A workstation includes special software and certain peripherals.

INDEX

A

Access management tools, 126
Advanced technologies (HCIT), 50–51*t*
Affiliation with central services IDS model, 69–71, 70*f*, 74*f*–75*f*
Affiliation IDS model, 62, 67*f*–68, 74*f*–75*f*
Antivirus software, 140
Application software, 137. *See also* HCIT application systems
ASPs (application service providers), 6

B

Bandwidth, 138
Business to Technology Alignment methodology, 84–85*f*, 92*f*

C

CD-ROM medical research tools, 3
CEO (chief executive officer): introduction to IT for, 136–138; technology knowledge needed by, 135–136
Cerner Corporation, 24
Certificate authority, 139
CID (contract issues document), 106
CIO (chief information officer): described, 112; emerging roles of, 115–116; management challenges of, 116–118; oversight and governance by, 118–120; responsibilities of, 114–115; role of, 113*t*
CKO (chief knowledge officer), 115
Claims management, 37
Client-server (C/S) architecture, 140–141
Clinical decision support systems, 40*t*
Clinical expert systems, 39, 40*t*
Clinical systems, 40–42*t*

CMIO (chief medical information officer), 115, 116
Competency development: information technology impact on, 2; IS department operational, 129–130; IS department political and strategic, 130–132; IT financial/benefits, 78–79
Computer telephony/interactive voice response technologies, 28
Computers: database tools used with, 138; described, 136; hardware/peripherals equipment of, 136–137; software used with, 137–138
Consulting IT services, 18, 21*t*
Consumer health record, 44
Consumer health systems, 49–50*t*
Core transaction systems: described, 31–32; Internet and e-commerce activity, 33, 35, 37; overview of individual, 32–33; as systems life cycle consideration, 84
Corporate ownership IDS model, 71*f*–72, 74*f*–75*f*
CSC, 24
CTO (chief technology officer), 115–116

D

Data collection tools, 98–100, 99*e*
Data exchanges: patient scheduling, 54*t*; return-on-investment (ROI) of HCIT, 52–53, 55; security issues of, 139–140
Data integration tools, 28
Data storing technology, 28
Database tools, 138
Decision support systems (DDS): described, 38–40*t*; systems life cycle and, 84

Digital certificate, 139
Disaster planning, 127–128
DLS (digital subscriber line), 138–139
DRGs (diagnosis-related groupings), 86

E

Electronic commerce (e-commerce): clinical systems and, 41–42t; consumer health systems and, 49–50t; core transaction systems running, 33, 35, 37; decision support systems (DSS) and, 38–40t; electronic medical records (EMR) and, 42–45; enterprise systems and, 48t; IS department management of, 125; managed care systems and, 45, 46t–47t; technology for, 28
Electronic mail (e-mail), 141
Electronic medical records (EMR), 42–45
Encryption, 139
Enterprise care model, 14–15
Enterprise systems, 47–48t
Extranet systems, 30, 31f, 142

F

Financial decision support systems, 39t
Firewalls, 140

G

General clinical systems, 41, 42t
General financial management systems, 32, 34t

H

Hardware: life cycle and price/performance of, 86–87; manufacturers of, 18, 20t
HCIT application systems: advanced technologies, 50–51t; benefit mapping of, 55, 56t, 57f; clinical, 40–42t, 43t; consumer health, 49–50t; core transaction, 31–37; decision support, 38–40t; electronic medical records, 42–45; enterprise, 47–48t; human resources, 38; managed care, 45, 46t–47t; return on investment (ROI) of, 52–55; types listed, 10t–13t; vendors supplying, 18, 19t
HCIT architecture: adding "Net" layers to, 30; client-server (C/S), 140–141; foundation technologies of, 28–29; Internet and, 29–30; Internet-intranet-extranet systems, 30, 31f, 142

HCIT firms, 23
HCIT (health care information technology): analysis using, 4; budget/expenditure issues of, 6–7; emerging importance of, 1; expansion issues of, 7–8; importance of planning, 3–4; multiple models of integration of, 5–6; myths and realities of, 2–8; overview of, 9, 10t–13t; range and capabilities of, 4–5; regulatory pressures on, 16–17; responsibility and vision of, 6; return on investment (ROI) of, 52–57f. See also IS (information services) department; IT (information technology)
HCIT investment: benefit mapping of, 55, 56t, 57f; return on investment (ROI) of, 52–55, 110
HCIT management. See IS (information services) department
HCIT market: diversity and amount of venders in, 22; evolution toward value-center services by, 23–24; public investment segment of, 23; supplier segment of, 17–18, 19t–21t; trends affecting providers in, 14–17; trends affecting supplier segment of, 22–24
HCIT suppliers: comparison of, 19t–21t; five subgroups of, 17–18
Health care executives: CEO (chief executive officer), 135–138; CIO (chief information officer), 112, 113t, 114–120; CKO (chief knowledge officer), 115; CTO (chief technology officer), 115–116; importance of IT knowledge by, 8
Health care providers: comparison of IT market, 19t–21t; trends affecting market of, 14–17
HIPAA (Health Insurance Portability and Accountability Act), 17, 47, 114
Home health care management systems, 33, 36t
Hospital industry: maturation of, 14; transition to enterprise care model by, 14–15
Human resources management, 38
Human resources systems, 38

I

IDS information technology management: of central/specialized IT governance bodies, 76; common and advanced challenges of, 79–82; using consolidation of systems, 78; of cultural implications of merger, 81–82; developing IT financial/benefits competency, 78–79; of disparate IT development levels, 79–80; of expanded organization, 80–81; of initiatives for IDS development, 77; of interim/long-range IT plans, 77; issues of, 73; structures of planning and, 73, 76–79

IDSs (integrated delivery systems): affiliation with central services model of, 69–71, 70*f*, 74*t*–75*t*; affiliation model of, 62, 67*f*–68, 74*t*–75*t*; components of integration in, 60–61*e*; corporate ownership model of, 71*f*–72, 74*t*–75*t*; defining integrated aspect of, 60; experimentation with, 5–6; functions of, 59; key applications and focus of, 62, 64*t*–66*t*; mixed approach to integration of, 62, 63*t*; regional delivery model of, 59, 68–69*f*, 74*t*–75*t*; summary of, 72–73, 74*t*–75*t*; "virtual," 72

Imaging systems, 29

Input devices, 137

Integrated medical devices, 29

Integrated system, 140

Intellectual property/ownership rights, 105–106

Interface software, 140

Internet: as change driver, 29–30; clinical systems and, 41–42*t*; consumer health and, 49–50*t*; core transaction systems running, 33, 35, 37; decision support systems and, 38–40*t*; described, 141; electronic medical records and, 43–45; enterprise systems and, 48*t*; impact on HCIT, 2; IS department management of, 125; managed care systems and, 45, 46*t*–47*t*. *See also* IT (information technology)

Internet-intranet-extranet systems: architecture of, 30, 31*f*, 142; software/service providers of, 18, 19*t*; technologies of, 28

IPAs (independent practice associations), 3, 59

IS department practices: "dot-com" phenomenon and, 132; operational competencies and, 129–130; political competencies and, 130–132; setting goals/objectives of, 128–129; strategic

competencies and, 130; vendor staffing issues of, 132

IS (information services) department: best practices of, 128–132; centralized vs. decentralized governance of, 119; CIO executive leadership of, 112; CIO responsibilities in, 114–115; defining, 111; disaster planning by, 127–128; emerging executive roles in, 115–116; governance committee responsibilities in, 119–120; information security/confidentiality issues for, 125–127; Internet/electronic commerce management by, 125; key functions and responsibilities in, 122, 124–125; management challenges of, 116–118; matching the CIO and organization, 112–113*t*; organizational structures of, 122; sample structure/responsibilities of, 124*e*; situational governance of, 121*t*; small delivery systems used by, 123*e*

ISPs (Internet service providers), 18, 141

ISSC (information systems steering committee), 76

IT (information technology): brief overview of equipment associated with, 136–138; complicated budgeting issues of, 6–7; current services/expectations of, 16; defining, 9; familiarity of CEO with, 135–136; systems life cycle and, 84, 87–88; telecommunications and networking, 138–141. *See also* HCIT (health care information technology); Internet

IT (information technology) infrastructure: life cycle and Internet-centric, 87; as life cycle track, 84

IT (information technology) planning: basic guidelines for, 93; factors to consider during, 89, 93; feasibility evaluation/market availability, 96–97; functions of, 88–89; going to action from, 94, 96; process milestones in, 93–94, 95*e*

IT value program, 78–79

J

JCAHO (Joint Commission on Accreditation of Healthcare Organizations), 114

JDBC (Java Database Connectivity), 138

L

LAN (local area network), 73, 77, 139
Life cycle. *See* Systems life cycle

M

Managed care systems, 45, 46*t*–47*t*
Medical management systems, 41, 43*t*
Medical profession IT acceptance, 2–3
Memory storage devices, 137
MIS (management information system), 111

N

Networking technology, 73, 77, 139
"Nursery cams," 35

O

ODBC (Open Database Connectivity), 138
On-line medical tools, 3
Original equipment (hardware), 18, 20*t*
Output devices, 137
Outsourcing IT models: life cycle and, 86; overview of, 18, 21*t*

P

Patient administration and management systems, 32, 33*t*
Peripherals equipment, 137
Personal health record (PHR), 44
Physician practice management systems, 32, 35*t*
Premier Health Alliance, 15

R

Regional delivery IDS model, 59, 68–69*f*, 74*t*–75*f*
Replacement IT market, 23
RFI (request for information), 98, 99*e*, 105
RFP (request for proposal), 98, 99*e*, 100, 105
ROI (return-on-investment): conducting an analysis of, 110; data exchange and, 52–53, 54*t*, 55; expectations of, 53*f*

S

Service providers: CID (contract issues document) from, 106, 107*t*; criteria for selecting IT, 102–103; negotiating favorable contract with, 103*e*–106

Software: antivirus, 140; interfaces, 140; overview of, 137–138
Software providers: data collection and analysis of, 98–100, 99*e*; importance of selecting, 97; requesting RFPs and RFIs from, 98, 99*e*, 100, 105; requesting VSP (vendor system proposal) from, 98, 99*e*, 101*e*; system life cycle and incentives of, 87; vendor demonstrations by, 100, 102
SQL (Structured Query Language), 138
Supply chain tracking, 37
System implementation: characteristics of structured, 106, 108; characteristics of successful, 108–109; components of plan for, 109*e*; conducting ROI analysis after, 110
System integration companies, 18, 21*t*
System utility, 138
Systems life cycle: Business to Technology Alignment approach to, 84–85*f*, 92*f*; four tracks of, 84; influences on, 86–88; information technology and, 84, 87–88; risks/considerations of, 88, 90*t*–91*t*; stages of, 83
Systems software, 137

T

Telecommunication technology, 138–141
Telecommunications/network services suppliers, 18, 20*t*
Three-tier client-server architecture, 141

U

University Healthsystem Consortium, 15
User education/training, 127, 131–132
User identification tools, 126

V

"Vaporware," 100
VHA, 15
"Virtual" IDS (integrated delivery system), 72
VSP (vendor system proposal), 98, 99*e*, 101*e*, 105

W

WAN (wide area network), 73, 77, 139
Web sites, 141
Workflow systems, 29